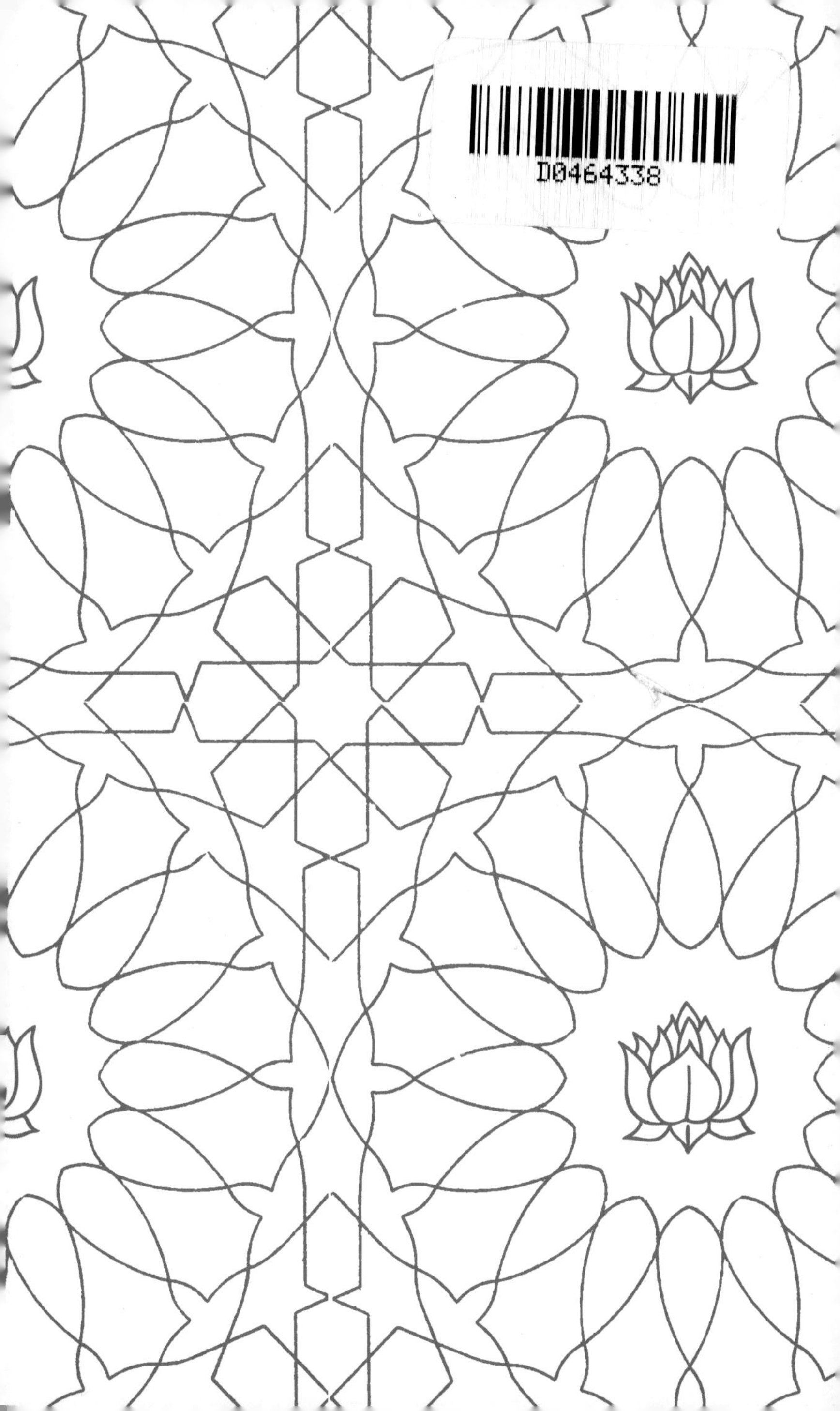
D0464338

THE ESSENTIAL DEEPAK CHOPRA SERIES

The Essential Ageless Body, Timeless Mind

The Essential How to Know God

The Essential Spontaneous Fulfillment of Desire

The Essential

Ageless Body, Timeless Mind

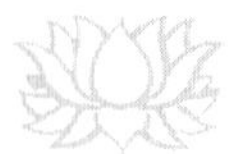

FUNDAMENTAL PRINCIPLES FROM THE ORIGINAL BESTSELLING BOOK

DEEPAK CHOPRA

The Essential

AGELESS BODY, TIMELESS MIND

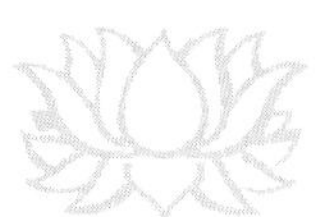

The Essence of the Quantum Alternative to Growing Old

Harmony Books *New York*

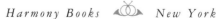

Published in the United States by Harmony Books,
an imprint of the Crown Publishing Group,
a division of Random House, Inc., New York.
www.crownpublishing.com

This is an abridged edition of *Ageless Body, Timeless Mind: The Quantum Alternative to Growing Old,* published in hardcover in the United States by Harmony Books, an imprint of the Crown Publishing Group, a division of Random House, Inc., New York, in 1993.

HARMONY BOOKS is a registered trademark and the Harmony Books colophon is a trademark of Random House, Inc.

Library of Congress Cataloging-in-Publication Data is available upon request

ISBN 978-0-307-40773-3

Printed in the United States of America

Design by Lauren Dong

10 9 8 7 6 5 4 3 2 1

First Abridged Edition

People don't grow old.
When they stop growing, they
become old.

ANONYMOUS

If you were to destroy in mankind the
belief in immortality, not only love
but every living force maintaining
the life of the world would at once
be dried up.

DOSTOEVSKY

I move with the infinite in Nature's power
I hold the fire of the soul
I hold life and healing.

RIG VEDA

Look at these worlds spinning
out of nothingness
That is within your power.

RUMI

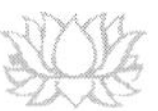

Author's Note

THERE ARE FEW THINGS IN LIFE THAT I FIND more gratifying than learning and teaching. We are all born with an insatiable curiosity about the world around us, and I was fortunate to grow up in a home that encouraged that appetite. Now, as an adult, I enjoy the best of both worlds: I can explore science, ancient wisdom, health, and spirit on the one hand, and on the other I can share what I've learned—helping others to satisfy their own curiosities—through my books and lectures.

When I speak to audiences, I find myself presenting my ideas in a manner that is concise or expansive depending on the length of time I have at my disposal. A five-minute segment on a morning television show requires a very different presentation from an hour on my weekly Sirius radio program, which in turn is very brief compared to one of the weeklong courses I teach around the globe. It occurs to me that the same holds true for what we read. After all, we don't always have the luxury of taking the time to explore the book-long articulation of a new idea, but we might have the time, say, to take in the essence of that idea.

It was from this thought that the Essential series was born. This series begins with three books that have attracted substantial followings in their expanded versions: *Ageless Body, Timeless Mind: The Quantum Alternative to Growing Old; How to Know God: The Soul's Journey into the Mystery of Mysteries; The Spontaneous Fulfillment of Desire: Harnessing the Infinite Power of Coincidence.* In these new essential volumes, I have distilled the most important elements from the full-length originals. It is my hope that this series will be of value to first-time readers of my work, as well as to those who may have already read these books, but wish to be inspired by these ideas all over again.

Ageless Body, Timeless Mind: The Quantum Alternative to Growing Old explores the astonishing parallels between the wisdom of Ayurveda, India's ancient system of mind-body medicine, and the counter-intuitive revelations of modern particle physics, when it comes to the subject of longevity. By drawing both from an approach tested by the passage of thousands of years and from research from the frontiers of modern science, we gain remarkable insight. Not only does it inspire us, but it also gives us practical strategies for harnessing the full powers of body, mind, and spirit. In the pages that lie ahead I believe you will find that not only can these techniques help you live longer, they will help you enjoy good health, mental acuity, high energy, and a positive outlook throughout your life. And that is my greatest hope for you.

I WOULD LIKE YOU TO JOIN ME ON A JOURNEY of discovery. We will explore a place where the rules of everyday existence do not apply. These rules explicitly state that to grow old, become frail, and die is the ultimate destiny of all. And so it has been for century after century. However, I want you to suspend your assumptions about what we call reality so that we can become pioneers in a land where youthful vigor, renewal, creativity, joy, fulfillment, and timelessness are the common experience of everyday life, where old age, senility, infirmity, and death do not exist and are not even entertained as a possibility.

Only our conditioning, our current collective worldview that we were taught by our parents, teachers, and society is preventing us from going there. This way of seeing things—the old paradigm—has aptly been called "the hypnosis of social conditioning," an induced fiction in which we have collectively agreed to participate.

Your body is aging beyond your control because it has been programmed to live out the rules of that collective conditioning. In order to create the experience of ageless body and timeless mind, which is the promise of this book, you must discard ten assumptions about who you are and what the true nature of the mind and body is. These assumptions form the bedrock of our shared worldview.

They are:

1. There is an objective world independent of the observer, and our bodies are an aspect of this objective world.
2. The body is composed of clumps of matter separated from one another in time and space.
3. Mind and body are separate and independent from each other.
4. Materialism is primary, consciousness is secondary. In other words, we are physical machines that have learned to think.
5. Human awareness can be completely explained as the product of biochemistry.
6. As individuals, we are disconnected, self-contained entities.
7. Our perception of the world is automatic and gives us an accurate picture of how things really are.

8. Time exists as an absolute, and we are captives of that absolute. No one escapes the ravages of time.
9. Our true nature is totally defined by the body, ego, and personality. We are wisps of memories and desires enclosed in packages of flesh and bones.
10. Suffering is necessary—it is part of reality. We are inevitable victims of sickness, aging, and death.

These assumptions reach far beyond aging to define a world of separation, decay, and death. Time is seen as a prison that no one escapes; our bodies are biochemical machines that, like all machines, must run down. This position, the hard line of materialistic science, overlooks much about human nature. We are the only creatures on earth who can change our biology by what we think and feel. We possess the only nervous system that is aware of the phenomenon of aging. And because we are aware, our mental state influences what we are aware of.

Each assumption of the old paradigm can be replaced with a more complete and expanded version of the truth. These new assumptions are also just ideas created by the human mind, but they allow us much more freedom and power. They give us the ability to rewrite the program of aging that now directs our cells.

The ten new assumptions are:

1. The physical world, including our bodies, is a response of the observer. We create our bodies as we create the experience of our world.
2. In their essential state, our bodies are composed of energy and information, not solid matter. This energy and information is an outcropping of infinite fields of energy and information spanning the universe.
3. The mind and body are inseparably one. The unity that is "me" separates into two streams of experience. I experience the subjective stream as thoughts, feelings, and desires. I experience the objective stream as my body. At a deeper level, however, the two streams meet at a single creative source. It is from this source that we are meant to live.
4. The biochemistry of the body is a product of awareness. Beliefs, thoughts, and emotions create the chemical reactions that uphold life in every cell. An aging cell is the end product

of awareness that has forgotten how to remain new.

5. Perception appears to be automatic, but in fact it is a learned phenomenon. The world you live in, including the experience of your body, is completely dictated by how you learned to perceive it. If you change your perception, you change the experience of your body and your world.
6. Impulses of intelligence create your body in new forms every second. What you are is the sum total of these impulses, and by changing their patterns, you will change.
7. Although each person seems separate and independent, all of us are connected to patterns of intelligence that govern the whole cosmos. Our bodies are part of a universal body, our minds an aspect of a universal mind.
8. Time does not exist as an absolute, but only eternity. What we call linear time is a reflection of how we perceive change. If we could perceive the changeless, time would cease to exist as we know it. We can learn to start metabolizing non-change, eternity, the absolute. By doing that, we will be ready to create the physiology of immortality.

9. Each of us inhabits a reality lying beyond all change. Deep inside us, unknown to the five senses, is an innermost core of being, a field of non-change that creates personality, ego, and body. This being is our essential state—it is who we really are.
10. We are not victims of aging, sickness, and death. These are part of the scenery, not the seer, who is immune to any form of change. This seer is the spirit, the expression of eternal being.

These are vast assumptions, the makings of a new reality, yet all are grounded in the discoveries of quantum physics made almost a hundred years ago. The seeds of this new paradigm were planted by Einstein, Bohr, Heisenberg, and the other pioneers of quantum physics, who realized that the accepted way of viewing the physical world was false. Although things "out there" appear to be real, there is no proof of reality apart from the observer. Every worldview creates its own world.

I want to convince you that you are much more than your limited body, ego, and personality. In reality, the field of human life is open and unbounded. At its deepest level, your body is ageless, your mind timeless. Once you identify with that reality, which is consistent with the quantum worldview, aging will fundamentally change.

ENDING THE TYRANNY OF THE SENSES

Why do we accept anything as real? Because we can see and touch it. Everyone has a prejudice in favor of things that are reassuringly three-dimensional, as reported to us by our five senses. Sight, hearing, touch, taste, and smell serve to reinforce the same message: things are what they seem. According to this reality, the Earth is flat, the ground beneath your feet is stationary, the sun rises in the east and sets in the west, all because it seems that way to the senses. As long as the five senses were accepted without question, such facts were immutable.

Yet Einstein and his colleagues were able to remove this mask of appearances. They reassembled time and space into a new geometry that had no beginning or end, no edges, no solidity. Every solid particle in the universe turned out to be a ghostly bundle of energy vibrating in an immense void.

From this perspective, it hardly seems possible that human beings could age at all. Weak and helpless as a newborn baby appears, it is superbly defended against time's ravages. If a baby could preserve its nearly invulnerable immune status, we would all live at least two hundred years, according to physiologists' estimates. A baby's cells are not really new—the atoms in them have been circulating through the cosmos for billions of years. But the baby is made new by an invisible intelligence that has come together to shape a unique life-form.

Aging is a mask for the loss of this intelligence. Quantum physics tells us that there is no end to the cosmic dance—the universal field of energy and information never stops transforming itself, becoming new at every second. Our bodies obey this same creative impulse. An estimated 6 trillion reactions are taking place in each cell every second. If this stream of transformation ever stopped, your cells would fall into disorder, which is synonymous with aging.

Day-old bread goes stale because it just sits there, prey to humidity, fungus, oxidation, and various destructive chemical processes. A chalk cliff crumbles over time because wind and rain beat it down, and it has no power to rebuild itself. Our bodies undergo the process of oxidation and are attacked by fungi and various germs. But we can renew ourselves.

In order to stay alive, your body must live on the wings of change. The skin replaces itself once a month, the stomach lining every five days, the liver every six weeks, and the skeleton every three months. By the end of this year, 98 percent of the atoms in your body will have been exchanged for new ones.

Einstein taught us that the physical body, like all material objects, is an illusion. The unseen world is the real world, and when we are willing to explore the unseen levels of our bodies, we can tap in to the immense creative power that lies at our source. Let me expand on the ten principles of the new paradigm in light of this hidden potential waiting beneath the surface of life.

1. There is no objective world independent of the observer.

The world you accept as real seems to have definite qualities. Yet none of these qualities means anything outside of your perception. Take any object, such as a folding chair. To you the chair isn't very large, but to an ant it is immense. To you the chair feels hard, but a neutrino would whiz through it without slowing down, because to a subatomic particle the chair's atoms are miles apart. Likewise, anything else you can describe about the chair can be completely altered simply by changing your perception.

Because there are no absolute qualities in the material world, it is false to say that there even is an independent world "out there."

All that is really "out there" is raw, unformed data waiting to be interpreted by you, the perceiver. In short, none of the objective facts upon which we usually base our reality is fundamentally valid.

A hundred things you pay no attention to—breathing, digesting, growing new cells, repairing damaged old ones, purifying toxins, preserving hormonal balance, converting stored energy from fat to blood sugar, dilating the pupils of the eyes, raising and lowering blood pressure, maintaining steady body temperature, balancing as you walk, shunting blood to and from the muscle groups that are doing the most work, and sensing movements and sounds in the surrounding environment—continue ceaselessly.

These automatic processes play a huge part in aging, for as we age, our ability to coordinate these functions declines. A lifetime of unconscious living leads to numerous deteriorations, while a lifetime of conscious participation prevents them. The very act of paying conscious attention to bodily functions instead of leaving them on automatic pilot will change how you age. Every so-called involuntary function, from heartbeat and breathing to digestion and hormone regulation, can be consciously controlled. The era of biofeedback and meditation has taught us that—heart patients have been trained in mind-body laboratories to lower their blood pressure at will or to reduce the acid secretions that create ulcers, among dozens of other things. Why not put this ability to use in the aging process? Why not exchange old patterns of perception for new ones? There are abundant techniques, as we will see, for influencing the involuntary nervous system to our advantage.

2. Our bodies are composed of energy and information.

To transform the patterns of the past you must know what they are made of. Your body appears to be composed of solid matter that can be broken down into molecules and atoms, but quantum physics tells us that every atom is more than 99.9999 percent empty space, and the subatomic particles moving at lightning speed through this space are actually bundles of vibrating energy.

The essential stuff of the universe, including your body, is nonstuff, but it isn't ordinary non-stuff. It is thinking non-stuff. The void inside every atom is pulsating with unseen intelligence. Geneticists locate this intelligence primarily inside DNA, but that is only for the sake of convenience. Life unfolds as DNA imparts its coded intelligence to its active twin, RNA, which in turn goes out into the cell and imparts bits of intelligence to thousands of enzymes, which then use their specific bit of intelligence to make proteins. At every point in this sequence, energy and information have to be exchanged or there could be no building life from lifeless matter.

As marvelous as this wealth of diverse intelligence is, at bottom there is one single intelligence shared by the whole body. As we age, this flow of intelligence becomes compromised in various ways. The specific intelligence of the immune system, the nervous system, and the endocrine system all start falling off.

Age deterioration would be unavoidable if the body was simply material, because all material things are prey to entropy, the tendency of orderly systems to become disorderly. But entropy doesn't apply to intelligence—an invisible part of us is immune to the ravages of time. Modern science is just discovering the implications of all this, but it has been imparted for centuries through spiritual traditions in which masters have preserved the youthfulness of their bodies far into old age.

In India, the flow of intelligence is called *Prana* (usually translated as "life force"), which can be increased and decreased at will, moved here and there, and manipulated to keep the physical body orderly and young.

3. Mind and body are inseparably one.

Intelligence is much more flexible than the mask of matter that hides it. Intelligence can express itself either as thoughts or as molecules. A basic emotion such as fear can be described as an abstract feeling or as a tangible molecule of the hormone adrenaline. Without the feeling there is no hormone; without the hormone there is no feeling. The revolution we call mind-body medicine was based on this simple discovery: Wherever thought goes, a chemical goes with it.

Medicine is just beginning to use the mind-body connection for healing—defeating pain is a good example. By giving a placebo, or dummy, drug, 30 percent of patients will experience the same pain relief as if a real painkiller had been administered. But the mind-body effect is much more holistic. The same dummy pill can be used to kill pain, to stop excessive gastric secretions in ulcer patients, to lower blood pressure, or to fight tumors.

Since the same inert pill can lead to such totally different responses, we must conclude that the body is capable of producing *any* biochemical response once the mind has been given the appropriate suggestion. The pill itself is meaningless; the power that activates the placebo effect is the power of suggestion alone. This suggestion is then converted into the body's intention to cure itself. Therefore, why not bypass the deception of the sugar pill and go directly to the intention? If we could effectively trigger the intention not to age, the body would carry it out automatically.

The decline of vigor in old age is largely the result of people *expecting* to decline; they have unwittingly implanted a self-defeating intention in the form of a strong belief, and the mind-body connection automatically carries out this intention.

Long before you get old, you can prevent such losses by consciously programming your mind to remain youthful, using the power of your intention.

4. The biochemistry of the body is a product of awareness.

One of the greatest limitations of the old paradigm was the assumption that a person's awareness doesn't play a role in explaining what is happening in his body. Yet healing cannot be understood unless the person's beliefs, assumptions, expectations, and self-image are also understood. Although the image of the body as a mindless machine continues to dominate mainstream Western medicine, there is unquestionable evidence to the contrary. Death rates from cancer and heart disease are provably higher among people in psychological distress, and lower among people who have a strong sense of purpose and well-being.

What the new paradigm teaches us is that emotions are not fleeting events isolated in mental space; they are expressions of awareness, the fundamental stuff of life.

Awareness makes a huge difference in aging, for although every species of higher life-form ages, only humans know what is happening to them, and we translate this knowledge into aging itself. To despair of growing old makes you grow old faster, while to accept it with grace keeps many miseries, both physical and mental, from your door. The commonsense notion "You're only as old as you think you are" has deep implications.

5. Perception is a learned phenomenon.

Perceptions of love, hate, delight, and nausea stimulate the body in extremely different directions. In short, our bodies are the physical results of all the interpretations we have been learning to make since we were born.

Your cells are constantly processing experience and metabolizing it according to your personal views. You don't just funnel raw data through your eyes and ears and stamp it with a judgment. You physically *turn into* the interpretation as you internalize it. Someone who is depressed over losing his job projects sadness everywhere in his body—the brain's output of neurotransmitters becomes depleted, hormone levels drop, the sleep cycle is interrupted, neuropeptide receptors on the outer surface of skin cells become distorted, platelet cells in the blood become stickier and more prone to clump, and even his tears contain different chemical traces than tears of joy.

This whole biochemical profile will alter dramatically when the person finds a new job, and if it is a more satisfying one, his body's output of neurotransmitters, hormones, receptors, and all other vital biochemicals, down to DNA itself, will start to reflect this sudden turn for the better.

There is no biochemistry outside awareness; every cell in your body is totally aware of how you think and feel about yourself. Once you accept that fact, the whole illusion of being victimized by a mindless, randomly degenerating body falls away.

6. Impulses of intelligence constantly create the body in new forms every second.

Creating the body in new forms is necessary in order to meet the changing demands of life.

As long as new perceptions continue to enter your brain, your body can respond in new ways. There is no secret of youth more powerful. New knowledge, new skills, new ways of looking at the world keep mind and body growing, and as long as that happens, the natural tendency to be new at every second is expressed.

In place of the belief that your body decays with time, nurture the belief that your body is new at every moment. In place of the belief that your body is a mindless machine, nurture the belief that your body is infused with the deep intelligence of life, whose sole purpose is to sustain you. These new beliefs are not just nicer to live with; they are true—we experience the joy of life through our bodies, so it is only natural to believe that our bodies are not set against us but want what we want.

7. Despite the appearance of being separate individuals, we are all connected to patterns of intelligence governing the cosmos.

You and your environment are one.

If you choose, you can experience yourself in a state of unity with everything you contact. In ordinary waking consciousness, you touch your finger to a rose and feel it as solid, but in truth one bundle of energy and information—your finger—is contacting another bundle of energy and information—the rose. Your finger and the thing it touches are both just minute outcroppings of the infinite field we call the universe. In unity consciousness, people, things, and events "out there" all become part of your body; in fact, you are only a mirror of relationships centered on these influences.

The possibility of experiencing unity has tremendous implications for aging, because when there is harmonious interaction between you and your extended body, you feel joyful, healthy, and youthful. Seeing ourselves as separate, we create chaos and disorder between ourselves and things "out there." We war with other people and destroy the environment.

What makes us old isn't the stress so much as it is the *perception* of stress. Someone who doesn't see the world "out there" as a threat can coexist with the environment, free of the damage created by the stress response. In many ways, the most important thing you can do to experience a world without aging is to nurture the knowledge that the world is you.

8. Time is not absolute. The underlying reality of all things is eternal, and what we call time is really quantified eternity.

Although our bodies, and the whole physical world, are a display of constant change, there is more to reality than process. The universe was born and is evolving. Before the instant of the Big Bang, time and space didn't exist as we know them.

The whole notion of time as an arrow shooting inexorably forward has been shattered forever in the complex geometries of quantum space, where multidimensional strings and loops carry time in all directions and even bring it to a halt.

The only absolute left to us is the timeless, for now we realize that our entire universe is just one incident springing forth out of a larger reality. What we sense as seconds, minutes, hours, days, and years are cut-up bits of this larger reality. It is up to you, the perceiver, to cut up the timeless any way you like; your awareness creates the time you experience.

9. Everyone inhabits a reality of non-change lying beyond all change. The experience of this reality brings change under our control.

At the moment, the only physiology you can maintain is time-based. However, the fact that time is tied to awareness implies that you could maintain an entirely different style of functioning—the physiology of immortality—which would correspond to the experience of non-change.

The "me" who is afraid of snakes learned that fear somewhere in the past. All my reactions are part and parcel of the time-bound self and its tendencies. Yet in a subtle way, we all sense that something inside us has not changed very much, if at all, since we were infants.

This changeless "me," whom the ancient sages in India simply called the Self, serves as my real reference point for experience. In unity consciousness, the world can be explained as a flow of Spirit, which is awareness. Our whole goal is to establish an intimate relationship with Self as Spirit.

10. We are not victims of aging, sickness, and death. These are part of the scenery, not the seer, who is immune to any form of change.

Life at its source is creation. When you get in touch with your own inner intelligence, you get in touch with the creative core of life. In the old paradigm, control of life was assigned to DNA, an enormously complex molecule that has revealed less than 1 percent of its secrets to geneticists. In the new paradigm, control of life belongs to awareness.

The billions of changes occurring in our cells are only the passing scenery of life; behind their mask is the seer, who represents the source of the flow of awareness. Everything I can possibly experience begins and ends with awareness; every thought or emotion that captures my attention is a tiny fragment of awareness; all the goals and expectations I set for myself are organized in awareness.

We are made victims of sickness, aging, and death by gaps in our self-knowledge. To lose awareness is to lose intelligence; to lose intelligence is to lose control over the end product of intelligence, the human body.

Therefore, the most valuable lesson the new paradigm can teach us is this: If you want to change your body, change your awareness first.

Our fearful images of growing old, coupled with high rates of disease and senility among the elderly, resulted in grim, self-fulfilling expectations.

Aging made sense in a scheme of Nature where all things change, fade away, and die. It makes much less sense in a world where an endless flow of ever-renewing intelligence is present all around us. Which view you adopt is your choice.

There is no limit to the energy, information, and intelligence concentrated in one person's existence. The emptiness at the core of every atom is the womb of the universe; in the flicker of thought when two neurons interact there is an opportunity for a new world to be born. This book is about exploring that silence where time's breath does not wither but only renews. Look to the land where no one is old; it is nowhere but in yourself.

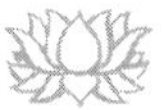

In Practice

How to Reinterpret Your Body

The first step toward experiencing your body in a different way is to change your interpretation of it.

Try to let go of the assumption that your body is aging because things just are that way. While still honoring your deep belief in aging, sickness, and death, allow yourself to set aside the old paradigm for a moment.

The quantum worldview, or the new paradigm, teaches us that we are constantly making and unmaking our bodies. Behind the illusion of its being a solid, stable object, the body is a process, and as long as that process is directed toward renewal, the cells of the body remain new, no matter how much time passes or how much entropy we are exposed to.

To have a renewed body, you must be willing to have new perceptions that give rise to new solutions. The exercises below are designed to help you open up new perceptions. Ideally, as we move on to later exercises, knowledge and experience will begin to fuse—that is the sign that you are fully assimilating this new worldview in place of the old.

Exercise 1: Seeing Through the Mask of Matter

The most important step in gaining the experience of ageless body is to unfreeze the perceptions that have locked you into feelings of isolation, fragmentation, and separateness. So let us see if we can go beyond the senses to find a level of transcendental experience, which is in fact *more real* than the world of the senses.

Look at your hand and examine it closely. This is the hand your senses report to you, a material object composed of flesh and blood. In this first exercise we will attempt to "thaw out" your hand and give you a different experience of it beyond the reach of your senses.

Holding the image of your hand in your mind's eye, imagine that you are examining it through a high-powered microscope whose lens can penetrate the finest fabrics of matter and energy. At the lowest power, you no longer see smooth flesh but a collection of individual cells loosely bound by connective tissue. Moving closer, you can see separate atoms of hydrogen, carbon, oxygen, and so on, which have no solidity at all—they are vibrating, ghostly shadows revealed through the microscope as patches of light and dark.

You have arrived at the boundary between matter and energy, for the subatomic particles making up each atom—whirling electrons dancing around a nuclear core of protons and neutrons—are not spots and dots of matter. At this level you see that all things you once took to be solid are just energy trails.

Now you start sinking even deeper into quantum space. All light disappears, replaced by yawning chasms of black emptiness. The blackness closes in, and you are in a place where not just matter and energy are gone, but space and time as well.

You have left behind your hand as a space-time event. There is no such thing as "before" or "after" in this region. You are everywhere and nowhere.

Has your hand ceased to exist? No, for in crossing the boundary of the fourth dimension, you didn't go anywhere; the whole notion of place and time simply doesn't apply anymore. All the grosser levels of perception are still available to you; your hand still exists at all these levels you have traversed—quantum, subatomic, atomic, molecular, cellular—connected by invisible intelligence to the place where you now find yourself.

Now examine your hand with a new understanding—it is the stepping-off point for a dizzying descent into the dance of life, where the dancers disappear if you approach too near and the music fades away into the silence of eternity. The dance is forever, and the dance is you.

Exercise 2: Closing the Gap

Now that we have touched that level of quantum space underlying all physical existence, I want you to become more comfortable there.

Imagine two candles standing about three feet apart on a table in front of you. To your eyes they appear separate and independent, yet the light they cast fills the room with photons; the entire space between them is bridged by light, and therefore there is no real separation at the quantum level. Now carry one of the candles outside at night and hold it up against a background of stars. The pinpoints of light in the sky may be billions of light-years away, yet at the quantum level each star is just as connected to your candle as the second candle in the room; the vast space between them contains waves of energy that bind them.

As you look at the candle and the distant stars, photons of light from both land on your retina. There they trigger flashes of electrochemical discharge that belong to a different vibratory frequency from visible light, yet they are part of the same electromagnetic field. Therefore, you are another candle—or star—whose local concentration of matter and energy is one outcropping in the infinite field that surrounds and supports you.

Think about this organic connection between everything in existence. The lessons of this exercise are

- No matter how separate anything appears to the senses, nothing is separate at the quantum level.

- The quantum field exists in, around, and through you. You are not looking at the field—in every wave and particle, the field is your extended body.
- Each of your cells is a local concentration of information and energy inside the wholeness of information and energy of your body. Likewise, you are a local concentration of information and energy in the wholeness that is the body of the universe.

Exercise 3: Breathing the Field

The quantum field transcends everyday reality, yet it is extremely intimate to your experience. To fetch a word from your memory, to feel an emotion, to grasp a concept—these are events that change the entire field.

At its finest level, every physiological process registers in the fabric of Nature. In other words, the more refined a process is, the more connected to the basic activity of the cosmos. Here is a simple breathing exercise that can give you a remarkably vivid experience of this phenomenon.

Sit comfortably in a chair with your eyes closed. Gently and slowly inhale through your nostrils, imagining as you do so that you are drawing the air from a point infinitely far away.

Now slowly and easily exhale, sending every atom of air back to its source infinitely far away. It may help if you envision a thread that extends from you to the far reaches of the cosmos; or you might visualize a star hovering in front of you that is sending light from infinitely far away—in either case, imagine the thread or the star as your source of air. If you aren't a good visualizer, don't worry; just hold the word *infinite* in your mind as you breathe. Whatever technique you use, the aim is to *feel* each breath coming to you from the quantum field, which at a subtle level is actually happening. Reestablishing the memory of your connection with the quantum field will awaken the memory of renewal in your body.

Exercise 4: Redefining

Having absorbed the knowledge that your body is not a sculpture isolated in space and time, redefine yourself by repeating the following statements silently to yourself:

I can use the power of my awareness to experience a body that is

Flowing	instead of	solid
Flexible	" "	rigid
Quantum	" "	material
Dynamic	" "	static
Composed of information and energy	" "	random chemical reactions
A network of intelligence	" "	a mindless machine
Fresh and ever-renewing	" "	entropic and aging
Timeless	" "	time-bound

Another good set of redefining statements:

- I am not my atoms, they come and go.
- I am not my thoughts, they come and go.
- I am not my ego, my self-image changes.
- I am above and beyond these; I am the witness, the interpreter, the Self beyond the self-image. This Self is ageless and timeless.

If aging is something that's happening to you, then basically you're a victim; but if aging is something you learned, you're in a position to unlearn the behavior that's making you age, adopt new beliefs, and be guided into new opportunities.

Life is awareness in action. Despite the thousands of hours of old tapes that program our responses, we continue to live because awareness finds new ways to flow. The positive side of awareness—its ability to heal—is always available.

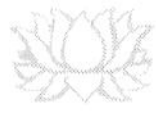

Learning Not to Age

The Link Between Belief and Biology

Although awareness gets programmed in thousands of ways, the most convincing are what we call beliefs. But unlike a thought, which actively forms words or images in your brain, a belief is generally silent. A person suffering from claustrophobia doesn't need to think, "This room is too small." Put into a small, crowded room, his body reacts automatically. Somewhere in his awareness is a hidden belief that generates all the physical symptoms of fear without his having to think about it.

People with phobias struggle desperately to use thoughts to thwart their fear, but to no avail. The habit of fear has sunk so deep that the body remembers to carry it out, even when the mind is resisting with all its might.

Our beliefs in aging hold just this kind of power over us. Let me give an example.

Daring gerontologists at Tufts University visited a nursing home, selected a group of the frailest residents, and put them on a weight-training regimen. Within eight weeks, wasted muscles had come back by 300 percent, coordination and balance improved, and overall a sense of active life returned. Some of the subjects who had not been able to walk unaided could now get up and go to the bathroom in the middle of the night by themselves, an act of reclaimed dignity that is by no means trivial. What makes this accomplishment truly wondrous, however, is that the youngest subject in the group was 87 and the oldest 96.

These results were always possible; nothing new was added here to the capacity of the human body. All that happened was that a belief changed, and when that happened, aging changed. If you are 96 years old and afraid to move your body, it will waste away.

Our notions of aging have been drastically modified over the last two decades. In the early 1970s, doctors began to notice patients in their sixties and seventies whose bodies still functioned with the vigor and health of middle age. These people ate sensibly and looked after their bodies. Although they exhibited some of the accepted signs of old age—higher blood pressure and cholesterol, and tendencies to put on body fat, to become farsighted, and to lose the top range of their hearing—there was nothing elderly about these people. The "new old age," as it came to be called, was born.

The new old age arrived on the scene after more than half a century of improved living conditions and intensive medical progress. The average American life span of 49 years in 1900 jumped to 75 in 1990. To put this huge increase in perspective, the years of life we have gained in less than a century are equal to the total life span that individuals enjoyed for more than four thousand years; from prehistoric times to the dawn of the Industrial Revolution, the average life span remained below 45. Only 10 percent of the general population used to make it to 65, but today 80 percent of the population lives at least that long.

One thing the quantified research has shown so far is very valuable: Biological age responds to psychological age. By nurturing your inner life, you are using the power of awareness to defeat aging at its source. On the other hand, changes of awareness in the direction of apathy, helplessness, and dissatisfaction push the body into rapid decline.

In 1957, Flanders Dunbar, a professor of medicine at Columbia University, reported on a study of centenarians and "nimble nonagenarians." She found that psychological adaptability in the face of stress was dominant among these people. Although everyone has occasions for grief, shock, sadness, and disappointment, some of us spring back much better than others.

For some, the journey of life, however harsh on the outside, is met with resilience instead of brittleness; they are the reeds who bend in the storm, not the oaks who stand stiff and break.

THE COMMON DENOMINATOR OF ALL ADAPTABLE people is that they actually work, on a daily basis, at keeping their awareness open. Most of this book is devoted to that work, and I feel that there is no higher life purpose than trying to open your awareness until the full impact of reality—in all its beauty, truth, wonder, and sacredness—is consciously experienced.

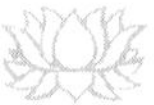

The Opening of Awareness

In our society we pick up hundreds of external cues about how to live, yet experience teaches us over and over that internal cues are the ones we must heed. Most people who age successfully follow their instincts, finding out what works for them.

The fact that successful survival is so individual is not an incidental factor—it is among the most important.

To gain control over the aging process, one must first be aware of it, and no two people share the same awareness. It is in the absence of being aware, when we don't see anything happening, that physiological processes slip out of our control.

As soon as you pay attention to any function, a transformation takes place. Every time you exercise your biceps, you are *teaching* it to be stronger, and your brain, lungs, heart, endocrine glands, and even immune system are adapting to a new mode of functioning. Conversely, if you move your body without awareness, passivity takes the place of learning. Biceps, heart, lungs, endocrine glands, and immune system eventually lose function instead of gain it.

Awareness, once it becomes conditioned, assumes the shape of habit; unconscious repetition reinforces the destructive patterns, and unless new learning takes place, inertia will carry the body downhill year after year.

In the following exercises, we will explore how to consciously call upon the power of awareness and use it to our benefit, for if we do not use it consciously, our awareness will be trapped in the old conditioning that creates the aging process.

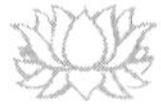

In Practice

Using the Power of Awareness

The exercises below are designed to prove that you can consciously direct the flow of energy and information in your body.

Below are some beginning procedures for localizing attention and fulfilling intentions. We will progress to deeper, more powerful techniques in later sections, but even at these stages, the connections being forged between mind and body are extremely helpful for breaking out of the old pathways that create aging.

Exercise 1. Paying Attention to Your Body

In this first exercise, you are asked to easily direct your attention to each area of the body; as this happens, the act of paying attention releases deep-stored stresses. Like a child, your body wants attention and feels comforted when it receives it.

SIT WITH YOUR EYES CLOSED IN A COMFORTable chair or lie down. (Choose a quiet room that is free of distracting noises.) Place your attention on the toes of your right foot. Curl them down until they feel tense, then release the tension and feel the sense of relaxation that flows into them. Don't rush either the tensing or the relaxing; take time to feel what is happening. Now let out a long, deep sigh as if you are breathing out of your toes, letting all stored fatigue and tension flow away with your breath.

Once you have this basic technique down, take your attention to all parts of the body in the following order. Remember that this is not just a muscle relaxation technique; your attention needs to linger comfortably at each bodily location.

Right foot: toes, top of foot, sole of foot, ankle (two stages: flexing back, then flexing forward)

Left foot

Right buttock and upper thigh

Left buttock and upper thigh

Abdominal muscles (diaphragm)

Lower back, upper back

Right hand: fingers, wrist (two stages: flexing back, then flexing forward)

Left hand

Shoulders (flexing forward, then flexing upward toward neck)

Neck (flexing forward, then flexing backward)

Face (screwing face into tight grimace, then tensing brow and forehead)

A complete circuit of the body as described above takes about fifteen minutes. If you are pressed for time, a short version involves only the toes, diaphragm, fingers, shoulders, neck, and face.

Exercise 2: Focused Intention

This exercise demonstrates that having an intention is enough to accomplish a result. When properly focused—which means easily and without strain—awareness has the ability to carry out quite specific commands.

In the procedure given here, you will experience the effortless way that intentions can get fulfilled, bypassing the ego and the rational mind (for best results, do exercise 1 as a warm-up, in order to bring your body into a receptive state).

1. Take a piece of string about twelve inches long and tie a small weight at the end to form a pendulum (a lead fishing weight, household washer, or one-inch bolt will work well). Hold the string in your right hand and brace your elbow on a table or the arm of your chair so that you can hold the pendulum steady. Sit comfortably and make sure that the pendulum is not moving.

Now look at the weight and project the intention that the pendulum move from side to side. Keep your attention on the pendulum and keep the intention firmly in mind, but make sure you hold your arm steady. In a few seconds you will be surprised to see the pendulum start to move of its own accord.

Now change your intention to direct the pendulum back and forth instead of side to side. Again see this motion in your mind's eye and easily hold it there. Typically, your pendulum will hesitate for a few seconds, move erratically, then take up the desired direction.

After watching it for a few seconds, intend for the pendulum to swing in a circle. Again it will pause, move erratically for a second or two, then move exactly as you visualized.

Exercise 3: A Trigger for Transformation

Every intention is a trigger for transformation. As soon as you decide that you want something, your nervous system responds to reach your desired goal. This holds true for simple intentions, such as the intention to get up and get a glass of water, as well as for complex intentions, such as winning a game of tennis or playing a Mozart sonata. In either case, the conscious mind doesn't have to direct every neuronal signal and muscle movement to achieve its goal. The intention is inserted into the field of awareness, triggering the appropriate response.

In the following exercise, you are asked to participate in a kind of internal time travel using a visual image from your past; the purpose is to experience how quickly your body adapts to this intention with feelings of renewed youthfulness.

SIT COMFORTABLY OR LIE DOWN WITH YOUR eyes closed. Pay attention for a moment to your breathing, easily following the rise and fall of your chest, feeling the air as it passes in and out of your nostrils. When you are relaxed, conjure up in your mind's eye one of the most wonderful moments from your childhood. It should be a vivid scene of joy, and preferably you should be the center of some activity.

Details are important; for that reason, intensely physical experiences are the easiest to use. Feel the air and sunlight on your skin; sense whether you were hot or cold. Observe colors, textures, faces. Name the locale and the people in your scene. Notice how everyone was dressed and acted. But most important, recapture the feeling in your body as you rose up to blend into and become that moment. By rejoining the flow of one magical instant, you trigger a transformation in your body, duplicating the body chemistry of that youthful moment. The old channels are never closed, they are only unused. Therefore, by changing the context of your inner experience, you can go back in time using the biochemistry of memory as your vehicle.

Exercise 4: Intentions and the Field

The new paradigm tells us that our underlying reality, the field, is continuous and therefore equally present at all points in space-time.

It is normal to have all desires be fulfilled if your awareness is open and clear. It takes no special act of providence to fulfill desires; the universal field of existence has been designed to operate for that purpose.

Whenever a desire comes true, the mechanics have certain similarities for every person:

1. A certain outcome is intended.

2. The intention is specific and definite; the person is certain about what he or she wants.

3. Little or no attention is paid to the details of the physiological processes involved. Indeed, paying attention to the details inhibits the flow of the impulses of intelligence that produce the outcome, slowing down or preventing success.

4. The person expects a result and has confidence in the outcome. There is no anxious attachment to a result, however (if you are anxious about falling asleep, for example, that prevents the very outcome you desire).

5. There is a self-referring feedback involved. In other words, every fulfilled intention teaches you how to fulfill the next intention even better.

6. At the end of the process, there is no doubt that the outcome was obtained by a definite, conscious process that extends beyond the individual to a larger reality.

To take advantage of this knowledge, you can use the following exercise with any desire. Gaining clarity about the mechanics of intention is the most important step in achieving anything.

1. Sit quietly and use any of the methods already given for relaxing your body and feeling calm inside.

2. Intend the outcome you want. Be specific. You can visualize the outcome or express it to yourself verbally.

3. Don't get bogged down in details. Don't force or concentrate. Your intention should be as natural as intending to lift your arm or get a drink of water.

4. Expect and believe in the outcome. Know that it is certain.

5. Realize that doubt, worry, and attachment will only interfere with success.

6. Let go of the desire. You don't have to mail a letter twice; just know that the message was delivered and your result is on the way.

7. Be open to the feedback that comes to you either inside yourself or from the environment. Realize that any and all feedback was elicited by you.

This last step is extremely important. Being so conditioned by the materialist worldview, all of us tend to look for material results. The feedback produced from an intention is capable of manifesting in unexpected ways, but some result is always produced, however faint.

It is helpful to remind yourself that you can rely on this approach because you are tapping into the fundamental nature of your physiology as it operates all the time: "My internal cues are my best feedback, and the more I respond to them, the more I will amplify the force of my intention to get the outcome I want."

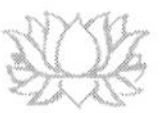

Defeating Entropy

THE BASIC MATERIAL OF THE HUMAN BODY IS extremely fragile. If you isolate a single cell and leave it outside on a balmy June day, it will wither and die in a matter of minutes.

The world is a dangerous place for life to survive in. A cosmic force stands ever ready to destroy life. It is called entropy, the universal tendency for order to break down into disorder.

The human body exists in utter defiance of entropy, since it is incredibly orderly and capable of adding to its order with even more complexity. Clearly, there is a counterforce pushing evolution along, creating life, fending off the threat of entropy.

The counterforce is intelligence. The two forces

are in constant battle. Creation and destruction co-exist.

Without destruction, life couldn't exist. Therefore, aging isn't simply the destruction of the body. As long as the body can renew itself according to its blueprint of orderliness, entropy is countered. As an old stomach or skin cell breaks down, it gets replaced.

We can call this balance of creation and destruction *dynamic non-change.* In other words, change takes place within a stable framework. As far as our bodies are concerned, this state of dynamic non-change is crucial. Tipping the balance in either direction spells disaster—lack of change leads to death; too much change leads to wild disorder (as when a cancer cell starts dividing indiscriminately until it eventually takes over vital tissues and causes its own destruction, along with that of the rest of the body).

Every cell knows how to defeat entropy by bringing intelligence to the rescue whenever disorder begins to intrude. The most critical example is provided by DNA itself, now known to have a remarkable capacity for self-repair.

You are talking to your DNA via the chemical messages sent from your brain, and these messages directly affect DNA's output of information. This knowledge raises the hope that the mistake of aging can be abolished at its source, in the depths of cellular awareness.

Like sharks roaming the cell, free radicals will attack almost any molecule; the extent of the damage they do is so wide that the free-radical theory of aging has grown in popularity with each passing decade.

EXERCISE: WORKING AGAINST ENTROPY

One of the simplest ways to prevent entropy is to give the body something to do. In physics, entropy is opposed by work, which is defined as the orderly application of energy. Without work, energy simply dissipates. Mental and physical neglect promotes premature aging. By now the value of regular exercise for all age groups has been well documented.

One special advantage exercise delivers is that it can reverse the previous effects of entropy. The major symptoms of biological aging can be improved through increased activity (the effect is boosted with secondary emphasis on improved diet).

The clear implication is that our notions about "taking it easy" as we age need to be reexamined.

THE VALUE OF BALANCE

Before you decide that hard work is the way to prevent aging, consider that "work" as defined by physics is not synonymous with sweat and strain. Work is needed to create orderliness and oppose the force of entropy. Exercise has a quantum effect, regardless of how much or little you do, by giving the body a chance to restore subtle patterns of functioning. Because the body uses both creation and destruction to keep its vital processes going, doing constant work is not the answer. Exercise has to be balanced by rest, because there is extensive muscle destruction during exercise that needs to be restored in periods of rest. In every area of life the key is balance, a very general term that can be broken down into four headings:

MODERATION
REGULARITY
REST
ACTIVITY

= BALANCE

Moderation means not going to extremes. Regularity means following a consistent routine. Rest means rest. Activity means activity. The cycle of rest and activity in lower animals is dictated by instinct, which humans are free to override. If we override it in the wrong direction, then we actually hasten entropy.

A balanced lifestyle is one of the most important steps toward retarding the aging process. What we want to do now is to probe into the deeper mechanics of balance to see if this beneficial effect can be improved. The secret of keeping destruction at bay is revealed only at the invisible level where intelligence is constantly preserving the balance of life.

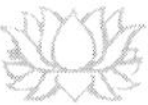

The Flow of Intelligence

Preserving the Balance of Life

Since all cells in the body are made up of molecules that found their place because DNA directed them there, it could be said that physiology is nothing but intelligence at work, and that every process under way in every cell is essentially intelligence talking to itself.

Being abstract and invisible, intelligence has to react before it can make itself known. Your brain makes its intelligence known by producing words and concepts; your body makes its intelligence known by producing molecules that can carry messages. It is fascinating to observe how these two types of intelligence meld into each other. The whole operation takes place at the quantum level, where the line between the abstract and the concrete blurs. At the source of intelligence there is very little difference between thoughts and molecules, as a simple example will demonstrate.

THE BODY AS INFORMATION

If you bite into a lemon, the juice instantly makes your mouth water as salivary glands under your tongue start secreting two digestive enzymes called salivary amylase and maltase. There is little mystery involved; the presence of food in our mouths automatically triggers digestion.

But what happens if you merely visualize a lemon or think the word *lemon* three times to yourself? Again your mouth waters and the same salivary enzymes are produced, even though there is nothing to digest. The message sent from the brain is more important than the presence of actual food. Words and images function just as well as "real" molecules to trigger the ongoing process of life.

By implication, the language we use to refer to ourselves is of tremendous importance. Child psychologists have found that young children are deeply influenced by ascriptive statements from their parents (e.g., "You're a bad boy"; "You're a liar"; "You're not as smart as your sister"). The mind-body system actually organizes itself around such verbal experiences, and the wounds delivered in words can create far more permanent effects than physical trauma, for we literally create ourselves out of words.

This is particularly important when we look at those two potent words *young* and *old.* There is an enormous difference between saying "I'm too tired to do that" and "I'm too old to do that." The first statement delivers a subliminal message that things will improve; if you are too tired now, your energy will come back and you won't be too tired later. Being too old sounds much more final, because in our culture, old is defined by the passage of linear time; old things don't become young again.

If we wanted to, we could transfer positive value to age. An Old Testament verse dating back to the reign of Solomon declares:

Gladness of heart is life to a man,
joy is what gives him length of days.

The belief that long life represents maximum joy is echoed in other cultures, particularly in those where reaching great age is esteemed and every added year holds more value.

If we look beyond the false duality of "old" and

"young," what we find is a different reality: The body is a network of messages constantly being transmitted and received. Life-nourishing experiences go far beyond cell biology.

The decisions we make in terms of our basic happiness and fulfillment are therefore exactly the ones that determine how we age.

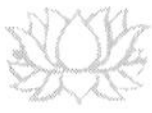

The Invisible Threat

Aging, Stress, and Body Rhythms

For more than fifty years physiologists have known that putting stress on an animal causes it to age very quickly.

Humans can withstand extraordinary stresses from the environment, but if we are pushed too far, our stress response turns on our own bodies and begins to create breakdowns both mentally and physically.

If someone points a gun at you and threatens to shoot, you instantly make a dramatic shift into a state of heightened arousal. A full-blown fight-or-flight response explodes throughout your body, preparing you for action.

Most of the time, your cells are occupied with renewal—roughly 90 percent of a cell's energy normally goes to building new proteins and manufacturing new DNA and RNA. When the brain perceives threat, however, the process of building is set aside.

As a temporary expedient, the stress response is vital, but if it is not terminated in time, the effects of catabolic metabolism are disastrous.

If the exposure to threat is not removed, arousal turns to exhaustion, because the body finds itself unable to return to the normal anabolic metabolism that builds reserves of tissue and energy.

Older people take longer to recover from stress, and they become less tolerant of strong stresses (for example, it is extremely rare for a young person to die of grief, an event that becomes more likely with age). One year of old age produces as much deterioration in the stress response as two years of middle age.

Whenever stress is blamed for an ailment, people jump to the conclusion that the problem is too much stress, but in fact the fault lies with the body's coping mechanism.

The theory of stress must be modified to include the mind-body connection, for such invisible elements as interpretation, belief, and attitude are enormously important in the actual workings of the stress response.

The totally personal way in which we filter all events determines how stressful they are. External stressors are basically triggers. If you don't feel triggered, there is no stress. A prevailing myth has arisen that some people thrive on stress. They perform best under high-pressure deadlines and blossom in the heat of competition. What's really happening is that they aren't being triggered physiologically.

Management of stress therefore turns out to be much more complicated than is generally supposed, because a person's interpretation of any situation is basically projected from his memory—our reactions to new situations are always colored by our experiences in the past. Instead of appraising each new situation afresh, we slip it into old categories. Neutralizing these old impressions is essential, for otherwise you have no control over stress—the stressful event will trigger your response automatically, making you its prisoner.

This unfortunate state has been extensively researched as that of "hopelessness/helplessness." Since growing old brings deep feelings of both kinds, this research has been extremely valuable. Laboratory animals can be induced to develop practically any disease through an application of stress. Or if a disease has been introduced, such as a chemically generated tumor, it can be made to advance much faster.

Induced stress in general has been found to hasten the spread of cancer in rats, rabbits, and mice, and to promote heart attacks.

THE CRITICAL FACTOR: INTERPRETATION

The effects of stress-producing situations vary enormously among different individuals. During the early years of the American space program, ground control personnel were astonished to discover that the heart rates of several astronauts showed no changes whatsoever as their rockets lifted off. Yet there are also hundreds of thousands of people who experience panic attacks whenever they fly in commercial airliners. Clearly, our interpretation of an event rather than the event itself is the critical component in our experience of stress.

One thing is certain, however. When a human being feels out of control, when for whatever reason there's a perception of stress, the body releases hormones identical to those associated with aging. This is a crucial point. Simply put, in order to ameliorate the process of growing old, we need to reduce the production of hormones that speed that process. We must recognize how our need for control gives rise to stress-producing interpretations of events, and we must instead embrace the wisdom of uncertainty and spontaneity. In our everyday lives, this wisdom is always available to us in many forms:

Laughter has enormous benefits both physically and psychologically.

Exercise stimulates the production of neurochemicals that create the experience of a "natural high."

Breathing loses its rhythm under stress. Two or three times a day, sit quietly, close your eyes, and gently place your attention on your breathing.

Music is a powerful antidote to stress, especially when it can be heard with full attention and enjoyment.

Visualization is simply the creation of an intensely pleasurable and relaxing experience in your "mind's eye."

Meditation can take many forms, including breathing awareness and primordial sound meditation, which uses a mantra as a tool for quieting the mind.

Sleep naturally reduces stress and restores internal balance. If you really need it, feel free to close your eyes at any time for a catnap.

Contact with the natural environment almost always reduces stress. Even if it's only buying a potted plant for your office or taking a brief walk in the park each morning, staying in touch with nature provides important stress-reducing benefits.

Relinquishing the need for control is the principle that underlies all genuinely effective stress-reducing techniques. If you begin to feel tense at any point during the day, remember that trying to master every detail of your situation is stressful and most likely counterproductive. Learn to relax and go with the flow of events.

In the laboratory, animals that are less evolved than rats (frogs, for example) do not respond to intangible stressors. The key factor is memory. If an animal has only a primitive memory, it won't recognize the difference between one situation and the next.

This has enormous implications for aging, because all of us carry around a world inside ourselves—the world of our past. We generate our own stresses by referring to this world and the traumas imprinted on it. There would be no stress without the memory of stress, for our memories dictate what frightens us or makes us angry.

Thus, stress becomes a self-fulfilling prophecy: Our reactions fit our expectations. The fact that every event cannot help but get imprinted with an interpretation gives memory its treacherous power.

MEDITATION LOWERS BIOLOGICAL AGE

Because the stress reaction can be triggered in a split second and without warning, it is impossible for us to control the molecules themselves. However, there is one mind-body technique that goes directly to the root of the stress response by releasing the remembered stresses that trigger new stress: meditation.

Before the early 1970s, these benefits were not even suspected. Meditation held little appeal for Western medicine until a young UCLA physiologist named R. Keith Wallace proved that besides its spiritual implications, meditation had profound effects on the body. The mantra meditation very quickly produced profound relaxation and significant changes in breathing, heartbeat, and blood pressure.

CONNECTING MIND, BODY, AND SPIRIT

Millions of Westerners wrongly assume that this makes meditation nonphysical, something you do in your head.

Unfortunately, our culture has made the mistake of deciding that the human body is a machine, an inert lump of matter that works without any intelligence of its own.

This kind of prejudice against the body runs contrary to the way that Nature fashioned us. Nature balanced mind, body, and spirit as co-creators of our personal reality.

When the material, psychological, and spiritual dimensions are brought into balance, life becomes whole, and this union brings feelings of comfort and security. Only if you feel sure of your place in the universe can you begin to face the fact that you are surrounded by creation and destruction as they constantly play themselves out. You cannot defeat entropy as a physical force, but you can rise to a level of realization that is not touched by entropy.

In the midst of change, there are five realizations that entropy cannot touch. They are expressed in every spiritual tradition and form the core of personal evolution age after age:

1. I am Spirit.
2. This moment is as it should be.
3. Uncertainty is part of the overall order of things.
4. Change is infused with non-change.
5. Entropy holds no threat because it is under the control of infinite organizing power.

These realizations are crucial because they allow a person to rise above the world of duality, which is inevitably caught up in the battle of creation and destruction. Let me translate each point in terms of the new paradigm.

1. I am Spirit.

Although my physical existence is confined to space and time, my awareness is not limited to that. Matter and energy come and go, yet all events are held together and made orderly by the deep intelligence that runs through all things. I am one aspect of that intelligence, an eternal presence of awareness.

A person who knows himself as spirit never loses sight of the experiencer in the midst of experience. His inner truth says, "I carry the consciousness of immortality in the midst of mortality."

2. This moment is as it should be.

This present moment is a space-time event within the eternal continuum. Since that continuum is me, nothing that can happen is outside myself; therefore, everything is acceptable as part of my larger identity. This realization is born when a person gives up his need to control reality.

In unity, every moment is as it should be. The shadow of the past does not spoil the fullness that is possible only in present time. The voice of inner truth says, "My desires are part of this moment, and what I need is provided here and now."

3. Uncertainty is part of the overall order of things.

Certainty and uncertainty are two aspects of your nature. At one level, things have to be certain or order couldn't exist. At another level, things have to be uncertain or there would be no newness. Evolution moves forward by surprising events; the healthiest attitude is to realize that *the unknown* is just another term for "creation."

In unity, a person sees the wisdom of uncertainty. He realizes that out of this total openness, order is still maintained. Opposites can and must coexist. The voice of inner truth says, "I embrace the unknown because it allows me to see new aspects of myself."

4. Change is infused with non-change.

Your desires and attentions guide the path of your growth. Because attention is always flowing, the dance never ends.

When you realize that you are held securely within this unchanging framework, the joy of free will arises. All possibilities are acceptable to the field, since by definition the field *is* a state of all possibilities. The voice of inner truth says, "I am getting to know the Absolute by playing here in the relative."

5. Entropy holds no threat because it is under the control of infinite organizing power.

Your body reflects the simultaneity of order and chaos. The molecules of food, air, and water swirling through your blood move chaotically, but when they enter a cell, they are used with precise orderliness. Chaos, then, is just a point of view. In unity, you realize that every step into decay, dissolution, and destruction is being used to organize new patterns of order. The inner voice of truth says, "Through alternating steps of loss and gain, silence and activity, birth and death, I walk the path of immortality."

THESE ARE DESCRIPTIONS ONLY; NO WORDS ON a page can substitute for the personal realization (what I have called the inner voice) as it unfolds for every individual. But it takes satisfying answers about who you are and why you are here to bring inner discontent to an end. In its true nature, life is comfortable, easy, unforced, and intuitively right.

This means that the self-realized state is the most natural one; the accumulation of stress, along with the aging that it produces, indicates that strain and discomfort are still present. The following "In Practice" section is devoted to ending this struggle by the technique that finally works—learning to accept your life not as a series of random events but as a path of awakening whose purpose is maximum joy and fulfillment.

In Practice

The Wisdom of Uncertainty

Life's uncertainty makes constant demands on everyone's coping mechanisms. There are basically two ways to cope with uncertainty—acceptance and resistance. Acceptance is healthy because it permits you to clear any stress as soon as it occurs; resistance is unhealthy because it builds up residues of frustration, false expectations, and unfulfilled desires.

In the following exercises you will learn how to restore your awareness to a state of acceptance, so that living in the present is as fulfilling as it can possibly be.

Exercise 1: Freeing Your Interpretations

Your life can be only as free as your perception of it. Whenever we look at a situation, we see our past in it.

If spiders frightened you as a child, you will project that fear onto spiders today. Just to realize that you are placing an interpretation on everything, no matter how trivial, is an important step toward freeing yourself from the past.

So it's important to question your interpretations. The only way you can end stress is by *perceiving* it to end. There's much more to say about how to accomplish this, but in my own life, I try to approach every stressful situation with the intention of defusing its threat in myself. Five steps have been immensely helpful:

1. Realize that you have an interpretation. In a conflict situation, I try to tell myself that my viewpoint is limited; I don't have a patent on the truth.
2. Set aside the old mindset. When I feel tense, I take this as a signal that I'm holding on too tightly to my point of view.
3. Look at things from a new perspective. I focus on the feelings in my body, and as I do, inevitably my mind starts to see things slightly differently.
4. Question your interpretation to see if it is still valid.
5. Focus on process, not outcome. Stress always

arises if you concentrate on how something *has* to turn out. I remind myself that I don't need to know where I'm going to enjoy the road I'm on.

When I go through these five steps, the daily annoyances that create inappropriate stress dissolve very quickly.

The exercise is to read and think about these five steps for changing your interpretations and then apply them. At first you should apply these techniques to a troubling event from your past. Think of someone who hurt your feelings very badly and whom you cannot forgive. The five steps might carry you into this line of reasoning:

1. I feel hurt, but that doesn't mean the other person was bad or meant to hurt me. There's always another side to the story, despite my hurt.
2. I've been hurt like this before, and therefore maybe I was too quick to judge this incident. I need to see each thing as it is.
3. I don't need to see myself as a victim here. When was the last time I was on the other side of the same situation? Didn't I feel pretty caught up in my own motives?

4. Let me forget my feelings for a second. How did that other person feel? Perhaps he just lost control or was too wrapped up in his own world to notice my hurt.
5. This incident can help me. I don't really care about blaming this person or getting back. I want to find out the kinds of things that create threat in me.

When you begin to get into the habit of consciously and carefully examining your old interpretations in this way, you create a space for spontaneous moments of freedom. These are the moments when your old mindset clears in a flash of insight. With that flash comes a sense of revelation, because you are looking into reality itself, not a reflection of your past. All the most valuable things in life—love, compassion, beauty, forgiveness, inspiration—must come to us spontaneously. We can only prepare the way for them (a spiritual friend of mine calls this "punching a hole into the fourth dimension").

Exercise 2: Peeling the Onion of the Past

The past is layered into us in many intricate layers. Your inner world is full of complex relationships, for it contains the past not only as it occurred but all the ways in which you would like to revise it. All the things that should have turned out differently do turn out differently in that place where you escape into fantasy, revenge, yearning, sorrow, self-reproach, and guilt. To get rid of these distractions, you need to realize that there is a deeper place *where everything is all right.*

In *Siddhartha,* Hermann Hesse writes, "Within you there is a stillness and sanctuary to which you can retreat at any time and be yourself." This sanctuary is a simple awareness of comfort, which can't be violated by the turmoil of events. It is the mental space that one seeks to find in meditation, which I believe is one of the most important pursuits anyone can follow. However, even if you do not meditate, you can approach this place of calm with the following exercise:

Write down this affirmation:

> I am perfect as I am. Everything in my life is working toward my ultimate good. I am loved and I am love.

Do not pause to analyze the statement, just write it down. When you come to the end, shut your eyes and let any response surface that comes to mind, then write down the first words that came to you (write this response directly under the affirmation). Your first thought is likely to contain a lot of resistance, even anger, because no one's life is perfect and it is hard to believe that everything is working out as it should. If your reaction shows similar emotion, it is an honest one.

Now, without pausing, write the affirmation again, shut your eyes, and once more write down the first words that come to mind. Do not stop to analyze or dwell on your reaction. Continue the exercise until you have repeated the affirmation and your response twelve times. You will be surprised at how much your reactions change; for most people, the final response will be much more positive than the first. Essentially, this exercise allows you to eavesdrop on the innermost levels of your awareness.

Most people have the highest resistance at the surface of their minds, because this is where their most public and guarded reactions operate. Going deeper, we hit levels of the most recent frustrations, wishes, and unreleased emotion. When you touch these layers, quite unexpected or irrational reactions can come out.

Deeper still are the layers where your most entrenched feelings are stored. If you feel basically unlovable, there could be a lot of pain and resistance at this level. But beneath even the most rigid conditioning, there is a layer of awareness that agrees without equivocation to the words "I am love."

This affirmation is extremely powerful for reminding yourself about your nature, but more than that, it reminds you of your purpose, which is to grow to the point where "I am love" is at the surface of your consciousness, not buried in the dark depths.

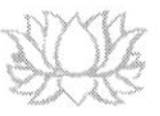

Longevity

I've never met Belle Odom, but I'm looking at her picture in the morning newspaper. She is a tiny old lady, smiling and waving a frilled lace handkerchief. Belle is in the paper because she has achieved the remarkable age of 109. Despite the fact that she is older than several states in the Union, her eyes look clear and alert; the accompanying article says that her mind is sharper than those of many younger residents at the nursing home where she lives.

The article rattles off some statistics about people who live to be 100 or more:

80 percent of all centenarians are women

75 percent are widowed

50 percent are in nursing homes

16 percent are black (the general population is only 12 percent black)

Belle is a black woman, born and raised in rugged Texas farm country. Until she turned 100 she lived alone in a cabin without running water; now she is the star resident of a Houston nursing home.

At 109, Belle has moved far beyond biological probability and into a mysterious and uncertain survival.

In the next few decades, barring a premature heart attack or a fatal disease or accident, you and I are likely to make it to 85 and 90.

The day you turn 50 is going to be your second birth. In all likelihood a complete lifetime lies ahead of you, lasting at least thirty or more likely forty, fifty, or even sixty years.

The great advantage of your second birth is that you can plan ahead. Your first birth was thrown at you, complete with total strangers who turned out to be your parents, an awkward, unformed body that had to be trained to perform the simplest tasks, and a bewildering world of chaotic sights and sounds your brain had to mold into something that made sense.

Fired by the possibilities of planning a whole new lifetime, I decided to take the opportunity seriously. I set aside all the stereotypes of old age that clutter the mind and approached my second birth (which is only four years away) with a wish list. What would I want should I live to be 100? Immediately the following desires came to mind:

I want to survive even longer, if possible.

I want to remain healthy.

I want a clear, alert mind.

I want to be active.

I want to have achieved wisdom.

As soon as I wrote down these desires, a surprising thing happened—they all seemed within my reach. I know what to do to be healthy today, and I can live tomorrow the same way. I've always been active, so why fear that I'll sink into a chair one day, never to get up again?

With this simple list I had turned survival from a threat into a desirable goal, because on my list were things I truly wanted.

There are societies where longevity is highly valued,

and it is there, in real-life settings, that we have found our best laboratory. We can examine a whole population who were instilled with that ambition from childhood on. The results have been remarkable.

SECRETS OF THE "LONG-LIVING"

Abkhasia, a remote mountain region of southern Russia, is a land of almost mythical old age. It is the only place I have ever heard of where there is a separate word for great-great-great-grandparents, which is applied only to the living. These were rural villagers, almost all of them illiterate field workers, who were reputed to have reached incredible ages of 120, 130, and upward of 170.

Although the region had suffered from malaria and typhus epidemics until the lowland swamps were drained by Soviet engineers in the 1930s, Abkhasia boasted five times more centenarians than any other part of the world, and 80 percent of the "long-living"—the word *old* was never applied to them—were active and vigorous. It was common for both men and women to work in the local tea fields for decades past the official Soviet retirement age of 60—champion tea pickers were given certificates when they reached 100.

For centuries in Abkhasia sedentary retirement was unknown except in cases of disability. Love of hard work was deeply ingrained among the Abkhasians, and records showed that a woman of 109 was paid for forty-nine full workdays in the tea fields one summer.

Favored with rich land and a climate suitable for corn, tomatoes, and all manner of truck produce, the population subsisted on home-grown vegetables and dairy products, with small amounts of nuts, grains, and meat to round out the fare. (Yogurt, a staple in their diet, has long had a reputation as a longevity food.)

Despite the fact that most of the long-living consumed cheese, milk, and yogurt every day, total intake of fat and calories was unusually low by Western standards, between fifteen hundred and two thousand calories a day.

As we in the West age, our bodies lose muscle mass and replace it with fat—at 65, almost half the body weight of both men and women is fat, double what it was in their twenties. By comparison, nearly all the long-living Abkhasians had lean physiques, with erect spines and firm muscles. Long after retirement, the oldest people thrived on outdoor life—they tramped up to the high grazing areas in summer and dug potatoes in their gardens. Even in cases where coronary arteries were blocked or other damage had occurred to the heart muscle, the walking and climbing in which everyone engaged seemed to offset physical limitation.

WHY WE NEED ABKHASIA

To me, Abkhasia was the place where the traditional concept of "old" never took root. The word was banished, and in its place the long-living pursued an ageless lifestyle—they galloped their horses, worked under the sun, and sang in choirs in which the youngest member was 70 and the oldest was 110. Abkhasia proved that growing older can be a time of *improvement.* Abkhasians toasted one another with the words, "May you live as long as Moses," and they venerated the long-living as people who were achieving an ideal.

By far the greatest advantage the long-living enjoyed was this: They trusted in their way of life. Abkhasians struck Western visitors as remarkably attuned to the rhythms of life, precisely what we have lost in this country.

One gets the sense of a people who have reached a

natural balance. Rather than struggling to break unhealthy habits, their culture had woven good health into their overall view of life.

In his book *The Methuselah Factors,* American author and Abkhasia scholar Dan Georgakas wrote, "Vegetables were picked just before cooking or serving, and if meat was to be part of the menu, guests were shown the animal before it was slaughtered. Whatever the food served, all leftovers were discarded, because they were considered harmful to health. Such concern for freshness guaranteed that a minimal loss of nutrients took place between garden and table. Most food was consumed raw or boiled, with nothing fried."

In every society, expectation rules outcome. In a culture where wealth is the highest goal, the entire society will focus on making money, prestige will accrue to those who make the most, and the poor will be regarded as failures. In Abkhasia, a great value was placed on longevity; therefore the entire society felt motivated to live up to that ideal. In America, the reverse is true; old age is not valued, much less exalted.

Huge differences divide the American and Abkhasian cultures. A lifetime of light eating and considerable physical activity is something we have to consciously learn again, but to fixate on those ingredients would cause one to miss the spirit of Abkhasia, which to me is far more inspiring as a motivation to survive to 100.

This country has recently experienced an unparalleled boom in centenarianism. The number of Americans who are 100 or over is currently estimated at 35,800—double what it was ten years ago and expected to double again before the year 2000.

We have won the struggle for longevity and now face the challenge of becoming a land where the long-living are still young.

SENILITY: THE DARKEST FEAR

Most of us would find it easier to bear the physical afflictions of old age than the mental ones. In India, where I grew up, age is still equated with wisdom. In the West, the longer one lives, the more one is suspected of mental incompetence. Alzheimer's has probably surpassed cancer for the dubious honor of being the most feared disease in America. I know 60-year-olds who obsessively pore over articles about Alzheimer's and panic whenever they forget a friend's telephone number, so convinced are they that contracting Alzheimer's is only a matter of time.

HOW THE BRAIN RESISTS AGING

Aging of the brain is not enough to cause Alzheimer's. Over time the structure of the brain is known to change. It grows lighter, for example, and shrinks slightly.

At present it isn't known why one old brain stays lively and creative—one thinks of Michelangelo designing St. Peter's when he was nearly 90 or of Picasso painting at the same age and Arthur Rubinstein playing the piano in Carnegie Hall—while another starts to deteriorate.

No two brain cells ever actually touch physically. They reach toward each other across a gap, or synapse, using hundreds or thousands of hairlike filaments called dendrites. One encouraging finding is that by remaining mentally active, older people may actually be growing new dendrites all the time.

This good news about the aging brain lifts our expectations that to keep one's faculties intact is completely normal. "Older people may not be as quick in timed tests," neuroscientist Robert Terry remarked, "but they don't lose judgment, orientation, or vocabulary. There is no way that people like Picasso, the cellist Pablo Casals, or Martha Graham could have continued to be so successful on half a brain."

Preserving intelligence in old age. The topic of aging and I.Q. provides a perfect example of how linear thinking misinterprets the complex changes that time brings. The human mind develops with experience along various lines. Brain studies help to indicate that organic changes keep up with the mind in its journey of expansion, but it is also important to trust the process itself, to realize that the mind *wants* to expand.

Psychologists are beginning to verify that human development extends into old age through higher states of awareness, that any decline in the brain's physical structure with age is offset by new mental accomplishments.

As the new old age obliterates the prejudice against old people, I believe we will witness a flowering of the visionary qualities that age can bring at its best. Vision is the hidden bond that unites youth and old age. In middle age we compromise our ideals in order to achieve success and security. The young are still impetuously idealistic, but the old can balance and enhance that through wisdom, perhaps the greatest gift of the human life cycle in its mature years.

THE LIMITS OF MEDICINE

Most people assume that medicine has been chiefly responsible for improving the health of old people and extending their life span; therefore, they look to doctors for cures for cancer, heart disease, Alzheimer's, and other degenerative disorders common to the elderly. This ignores the fact that successful aging is far more than the avoidance of disease, although that is important. It involves a lifelong commitment to oneself every day; a doctor can assist in making this commitment, but medicine is not a surrogate for it.

Longevity is still an individual achievement; it comes primarily to those whose expectations are high enough to reach for it. America could become a land where no one ever grows feeble and crippled by age, but for that to happen, we need to see the entire human life cycle as a rising curve. Today, fortunately, few "normal" signs of aging have gone unchallenged, and major studies have proved that we have expected far too little of the aging body, which holds great potential for improvement at very advanced ages.

NOT OLDER, BETTER

Everyone grows more unique with age, and that uniqueness includes the possibility for improvement on any front.

The new paradigm tells us that we are constantly making and unmaking our bodies at the quantum level, which means that we are constantly unfolding hidden potential. If we consider how to improve physical and mental function every day for the rest of our lives, three values emerge that must be part of everyone's intention:

1. longevity itself, since life is a primary good
2. creative experience, which keeps life interesting and makes us want more of it
3. wisdom, which is the collective reward of long life

It's impossible to set limits on what can be achieved in each area. Creativity and wisdom inspired Picasso, Shaw, Michelangelo, Tolstoy, and other long-lived geniuses to the day they died.

Psychologists who study creativity say that artists and writers often can produce more new ideas in their sixties or seventies than in their twenties. One interesting variable is that the later you take up any creative pursuit, the more likely you are to pursue it into old age.

Active mastery means having autonomy over one's life and circumstances, not power over others.

The most meaningful thing you can live for is to reach your full potential.

These latent potentials are closed off to the vast majority of people, who barely have skills to fill sixty-five years of existence. Therefore, it is extremely important to begin to develop your skills consciously, breaking free of social expectation and setting yourself the goal of becoming a master. To help you carve out your own ideal life, I have listed ten *keys to active mastery.* They summarize much of what we have learned so far about aging and awareness. They are also meant to be practical ideals, ones you can aspire to in action every day.

Ten Keys to Active Mastery

1. Listen to your body's wisdom, which expresses itself through signals of comfort and discomfort. When choosing a certain behavior, ask your body, "How do you feel about this?" If your body sends a signal of physical or emotional

distress, watch out. If your body sends a signal of comfort and eagerness, proceed.

2. Live in the present, for it is the only moment you have. Keep your attention on what is here and now; look for the fullness in every moment. Accept what comes to you totally and completely so that you can appreciate it, learn from it, and then let it go. Don't struggle against the infinite scheme of things; instead, be at one with it.

3. Take time to be silent, to meditate, to quiet the internal dialogue. In moments of silence, realize that you are recontacting your source of pure awareness. Pay attention to your inner life so that you can be guided by intuition rather than externally imposed interpretations of what is or isn't good for you.

4. Relinquish your need for external approval. You alone are the judge of your worth, and your goal is to discover infinite worth in yourself, no matter what anyone else thinks. There is great freedom in this realization.

5. When you find yourself reacting with anger or opposition to any person or circumstance,

realize that you are only struggling with yourself. When you relinquish this anger, you will be healing yourself and cooperating with the flow of the universe.

6. Know that the world "out there" reflects your reality "in here." The people you react to most strongly, whether with love or hate, are projections of your inner world. What you most hate is what you most deny in yourself. What you most love is what you most wish for in yourself. Use the mirror of relationships to guide your evolution. The goal is total self-knowledge. When you achieve that, what you most want will automatically be there, and what you most dislike will disappear.

7. Shed the burden of judgment—you will feel much lighter. Judgment imposes right and wrong on situations that just are. In judging others, you reflect your lack of self-acceptance. Remember that every person you forgive adds to your self-love.

8. Don't contaminate your body with toxins, either through food, drink, or toxic emotions. The health of every cell directly contributes to

your state of well-being, because every cell is a point of awareness within the field of awareness that is you.

9. Replace fear-motivated behavior with love-motivated behavior. Fear is the product of memory, which dwells in the past. Trying to impose the past on the present will never wipe out the threat of being hurt. That happens only when you find the security of your own being, which is love.

10. Understand that the physical world is just a mirror of a deeper intelligence. Intelligence is the invisible organizer of all matter and energy, and you share in the organizing power of the cosmos. Living in balance and purity is the highest good for you and the Earth.

LIFE IS A CREATIVE ENTERPRISE. THERE ARE many levels of creation and therefore many levels of possible mastery. Active mastery is not just a way to survive to extreme old age—it is the road to freedom.

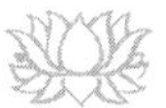

In Practice

Breath of Life

In its most complete sense, active mastery means handling the whole of life. It is a process of integration, for ordinarily many aspects of the mind are quite separate from and out of tune with the body, and both are separate from spirit.

Bringing all these ingredients back into unity isn't possible on either the mental level or the physical level alone. Paying attention to one automatically tends to exclude the other. Unity can be accomplished at very deep levels of awareness through meditation, when the duality of mind and body is transcended, but meditation is restricted to the special time set aside for it. How do we integrate the remaining hours of our active daily lives?

Thousands of years ago the ancient Indian sages

gave an answer in the form of *Prana,* the subtlest form of biological energy. Prana is present in every mental and physical event; it flows directly from spirit, or pure awareness, to bring intelligence and consciousness to every aspect of life. The critical importance of life energy has been recognized in many cultural traditions; the Chinese know it as *Chi* and control its flow through acupuncture, meditation, and specialized exercises such as tai chi. Other names for the breath of life appear in Sufism, mystic Christianity, and the teachings of ancient Egypt. What is universally agreed on is that the more Prana you have, the more vital your mental and bodily processes.

Depleted Prana is directly linked to aging and death. Nothing can remain alive when Prana is absent, because Prana is intelligence and consciousness, the two vital ingredients that animate physical matter.

In India the body is perceived first as a product of consciousness and only secondarily as a material object. Conserving Prana is considered extremely important.

Thus, a healthy life, as measured by the conservation of Prana, demands the following:

- Fresh food
- Pure water and air

- Sunlight
- Moderate exercise
- Balanced, refined breath
- Nonviolent behavior and a reverence for life
- Loving, positive emotions; free expression of emotion

Think of the difference between a salad fresh-picked from your garden and one made from the same vegetables bought in the supermarket. Contrast a picnic in the mountains with lunch at a hamburger stand. Freshness indicates the presence of Prana; staleness indicates its absence.

The factor least understood in our culture is balanced breath, which in India is considered the most important. Breath is the junction point between mind, body, and spirit. Every change of mental state is reflected in the breath and then in the body.

The various systems of Yoga in India teach many kinds of highly controlled breathing exercises, known as *Pranayama,* to balance the breath, but their actual goal is not to produce controlled or disciplined breathing under ordinary circumstances. Rather, paying attention to the breath is a vehicle for releasing stress and allowing the body to find its own balance. Once in balance, yogic breathing is spontaneous and refined, so that the refined emotions of love and devotion can be carried throughout the body at all levels. When your cells experience the fullness of Prana, they are receiving the physical equivalent of these emotions.

The following two exercises are for balancing your breathing. When properly done, these exercises will give you the experience of Prana as a light, sparkling, flowing sensation in your body. Mentally, balanced breathing is reflected in a sense of calm, lack of tension, and quietness, as the static of restless thinking gives way to silence.

Exercise 1: Body Breathing

Sit still in a chair listening to soft music, or outside listening to the wind in the treetops. As you listen, gently let your attention flow out of your ears as you easily exhale. Repeat for a minute, then do the same thing through your eyes, letting your attention go outward on the breath, slowly and gently. Repeat this through the nostrils, the mouth, then sit quietly just listening to the music with your whole body.

Now allow your attention to sink into your chest. Feel where your heart center is (at the point where the breastbone and ribs join) and breathe out through it, letting your attention go with the breath. Continue gently for another minute, then sit quietly, aware of your body.

This exercise consciously links respiration and the nervous system, helping to promote their smooth integration. Feeling your awareness as it flows out on your breath gives you a powerful sense of being at harmony with Nature.

Exercise 2: The Expanding Light

Stand in your stocking feet with your eyes closed, arms down at your sides, and vividly relive the sensation of your last exhilarating experience. Recapture the feeling of being happy, vibrant, and carefree.

As you do this, inhale slowly through your nose and begin to spread your arms out slowly. Imagine that as you inhale, your breath is expanding from the center of your chest. It is an expanding light that makes your arms float effortlessly open, and as the light expands, your happy, exhilarated feeling expands with it. Let the light grow as slowly or quickly as it wants, spreading from the center of your heart, reaching out to the tips of your fingers, up to your head, and down to your toes. You'll also be smiling, so let that grow, too.

At the point of maximum extension, start slowly exhaling through your nose and bring your arms back down to your sides. Do this slowly, taking longer to exhale than to inhale. Take the expanded feeling/light back down into your chest, until it is small and localized in your heart again. As your arms come back down to your sides, let your head drop forward.

Now repeat the exercise on the next breath, expanding the feeling again—don't pay attention to your physical movements, but stay with the feeling. You want to open and close it like a flower with each breath.

You'll notice that this is an extremely pleasant exercise, because as you open, your body fills with breath, awareness, and enjoyment all at once—the sensation is light, warm, tingling. As you close, the body relaxes and slumps under its own weight, becoming more grounded and still. You are exploring a complete range of feeling, which allows the subtle breath to penetrate into every channel.

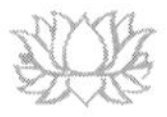

Breaking the Spell of Mortality

The ultimate boundary to human life is death, and for thousands of years we have tried to travel beyond that boundary. Despite the obvious mortality of our bodies, moments arise when the clear perception of immortality shines through.

Some people seem to have contacted this timeless realm through near-death experiences, but it is also accessible in everyday life.

Our first world is the world of action and activity and doing. But like flashes of spiritual lightning, there are moments when the second world makes itself known, full of peace and joy and a clear, unforgettable sense of who we really are. If the second world is inside us, so is the first, because everything to be seen, felt, and touched in the world is knowable only as firings of neuronal signals inside our brains. It all happens in here.

The first world contains sickness, aging, and death as inevitable parts of the scenery; in the second world, where there is only pure being, these are totally absent. Therefore, finding this world within ourselves and experiencing it, even for a moment, could have a profound effect on the process of sickness and aging, if not death itself.

The new paradigm assures us that there is a level of Nature where time dissolves, or, to turn it around, where time is created.

It has taken three generations for the new paradigm to show us that Being is a very real state, existing beyond change and death, a place where the laws of Nature that govern change are overturned. Death is ultimately just another transformation, from one configuration of matter and energy to another. But unless you can stand outside the arena of change, death represents an end point, an extinction. To escape death ultimately means escaping the worldview that gives death its terrible sense of closure and finality.

When the spell of mortality is broken, you can release the fear that gives death its power. By seeing through the fear you can turn it into a positive force.

"Let your fear of death motivate you to examine your true worth and to have a dream for your own life," Dr. David Viscott encouraged. "Let it help you value the moment, act on it, and live in it."

I want to go even further and suggest that when you see yourself in terms of timeless, deathless Being, every cell awakens to a new existence. True immortality can be experienced here and now, in this living body. This is the experience of timeless mind and ageless body that the new paradigm has been preparing us for.

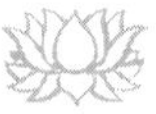

The Metabolism of Time

One of Einstein's brilliant contributions to modern physics was his intuition that linear time, along with everything happening in it, is superficial.

Einstein displaced linear time with something much more fluid—time that can contract and expand, slow down or speed up. He often compared this to subjective time, for he noted that spending a minute sitting on a hot stove seems like an hour, while spending an hour with a beautiful girl seems like a minute. What he meant by this is that time depends on the situation of the observer.

We all have a sense that time expands and contracts, seeming to drag one moment and race the next, but what is our constant, our absolute? I believe it is "me," our core sense of self. If you're bored, time hangs heavy; if you're desperate, time's running out; if you're exhilarated, time flies; when you're in love, time stands still. Time, in the subjective sense, is a mirror.

All of us, however, feel the pressure of a serious, threatening deadline over which we have no control—death itself. The attitude that life is a blossoming, not a race, can be achieved. But to do that, you can't believe that time is running out. Sending that message to your body's cells is the same, ultimately, as programming them to age and die. Yet the fact is that linear time *is* moving inexorably forward, and to overcome that, we must find a place where a different kind of time, or no time, can be experienced and internalized.

TIME-BOUND VERSUS TIMELESS AWARENESS

Throughout this book I've argued that how you age depends on how you metabolize your experience. And in the final analysis, how you metabolize time is the most important aspect of this process, because time is the most fundamental experience.

It's possible to have actual experiences of timelessness, and when that happens, there is a shift from time-bound awareness to timeless awareness.

Time-bound awareness is defined by:

- External goals (approval from others; material possessions; salary; climbing the ladder of professional success)
- Deadlines and time pressure
- Self-image built up from past experiences
- Lessons learned from past hurts and failures
- Fear of change, fear of death
- Distraction by past and future (worries, regrets, anticipations, fantasies)
- Longing for security
- Selfishness, limited point of view (typical motivation: "What's in it for me?")

Timeless awareness is defined by:

- Internal goals (happiness; self-acceptance; creativity; satisfaction that one is doing one's best at all times)
- Freedom from time pressure; sense that time is abundant and open-ended
- Little thought of self-image; action focused on the present moment
- Reliance on intuition and leaps of imagination

- Detachment from change and turmoil; no fear of death
- Positive experiences of Being
- Selflessness; altruism; sense of shared humanity
- Sense of personal immortality

Although I have described them as opposites, there is in fact a whole range of experience running from completely time-bound to completely timeless awareness.

MOST PEOPLE HAVE VERY LITTLE NOTION OF how much effort they expend to keep themselves trapped in time-bound awareness. In their natural state, both body and mind attempt to discharge negative energies as soon as they are felt. A baby cries when it is hungry, thrashes when it chafes, and falls asleep when it becomes exhausted. Once you reach adulthood, however, spontaneous expression has largely been squelched in favor of behavior that is safe, socially acceptable, calculated to get what you want, or simply habitual. This loss of spontaneity is a result of not living in the present, which I discussed earlier. But there is another result I haven't discussed: the loss of timelessness.

When the human organism is discharging its negative experiences efficiently, the mind is empty of past or future concerns; there is no worry, anticipation, or regret. This means that the mind is left open to Being, the simplest state of awareness. Unfortunately, normal life is far from this state. We are all time-bound, and only on the rarest occasions—generally when we least expect it—do we manage to break in to a conscious experience of our true nature.

The sense of freedom, of throwing away the old baggage, arises automatically once a person stops relating only to his limited self.

In moments of deepest awareness we completely transcend self-image. Paradoxically, this is when the spiritual masters say the Self is truly experienced, for the total absence of self-image leaves pure selfhood exposed. Compared to the rigidity of your ordinary sense of "I," the Self is a living, flowing sense of identity that is never exhausted. It is a state beyond change, no matter whether you experience it as a baby, a child, a young adult, or an old man.

Time-based existence isn't whole and never can be, because it is by definition made of fragments.

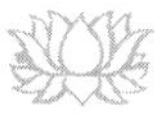

The Spell of Mortality

Overcoming the Illusion of Death

THIS SENSE OF BEING ONE WITH THINGS brings safety and the absence of threat. If harboring threat inside us is what gives rise to aging, then we cannot afford to live with our present fear of death. In actuality, death is not the all-powerful force our fear tells us it is. In Nature, death is part of the larger cycle of birth and renewal. This year's seeds sprout, grow, blossom, and set next year's seeds. The cycles of endless renewal are not beyond death—they incorporate death, using it for a larger purpose. The same is true inside our bodies. Many cells undergo aging and death as a choice, not because they have been forced into extinction by the grim reaper.

IN THE GRIP OF ILLUSION

To break free of the grip of death, you need to see that it is based on a very selective view of reality that was conditioned into you before you had a conscious choice.

The moment you confronted death, some psychologists argue, you bought into a notion that has gripped humanity for centuries. Your belief in death as an extinction doomed your body to decay, age, and die, just as did so many before you in exactly the same way.

It isn't death that hurts us but the dread of its inevitability. You may think that death is an awful event awaiting you in the future, when in actuality parts of your body are dying every second. Your stomach lining dies partially every time you digest food, only to be replaced by new tissue. The same is true of your skin, hair, toenails, blood cells, and every other tissue.

You may assume that death is your enemy, but all these cells are dying in order to keep you alive. If your stomach lining didn't die and get replaced over and over, gastric juices would sear a hole in your stomach wall after a few hours, and then all of you would die. The line between what is living and what is dead gets very blurry the closer you look. Muscles have a faster metabolism than fat; brain, heart, and liver cells rarely if ever duplicate after birth, while stomach, skin, and blood cells replace themselves in a matter of days, weeks, and months.

Some people recoil from all this talk about death, denying any interest in it. They don't fear death, they say, or if they do, it doesn't haunt them or hold the kind of power over them I have been describing. But unconscious forces are at work in us. We may all concede that we are going to die, but except in moments when we have to be present with the dead or dying, our dread is kept under wraps.

The fact that we all protect ourselves from dread doesn't mean that we have control over it. From within its dark pit, fear is still exerting control over us.

The point is not that death is a fiction, but that our belief in death creates limitations where none need exist.

THE USES OF DYING

One assumption we all tend to make is that death is somehow unnatural and, by implication, evil. I cannot agree. Nature is very tolerant and flexible about how death is used, or not used; and in the larger picture, questions of good and evil tend to look rather arbitrary. If you consider how life operates from the genetic level, DNA long ago discovered the secret of creating ageless cells. The hydra, for example, is a primitive water animal that can grow new cells as fast as old ones are shed. The hydra is always growing at one end and dying at the other, renewing its entire body every two weeks. This is creation and destruction in perfect balance, leaving no room for death.

Even among higher organisms, DNA exerts considerable control over death. The common honeybee, for example, can change its age at will. Every beehive needs young workers whose job is to stay indoors to feed and care for newly hatching larvae. After three weeks, these workers grow up and move on to become mature foragers, the bees who fly from the hive to collect pollen from flowers.

At any given period, however, there may be too many young workers or too many old foragers. In the spring so many new larvae may be hatching that the hive lacks mature foragers and needs more very quickly. When that happens, some of the young workers age into foragers in one week instead of the usual three and fly off seeking food.

With only slight changes, one could adopt this model for the human body: It is a mammoth hive of

50 trillion cells that grow old or stay young according to what is needed by the whole colony at any given moment.

How, then, can we learn to live within this continuity that is the wholeness of life? What about a parent's emotional devastation when a child dies, or a wife's when she loses her husband?

These feelings are natural, of course. But the pain does not have to be deep and enduring if you have absorbed the reality of life as an eternal flow in which there is no loss or gain, only transformation. In one of his sonnets Shakespeare wrote, "I weep to have what I fear to lose"—this is the inevitable result of attachment to time-bound awareness. The new paradigm holds that awareness is the source of reality, and two wholly different kinds of reality result from time-bound and timeless awareness.

All of us experience aspects of both realities, because our awareness is fluid. This flexibility is the true genius of human awareness, because it leaves all possibilities open. Yet obviously there are great advantages to living permanently in timeless awareness.

Humans are not trapped in time, squeezed into the volume of a body and the span of a lifetime. We are voyagers on the infinite river of life.

Immortality dawns when you realize that you deserve your place in the eternal flow. Nature waits to lavish this supreme gift upon you. Having nourished us for millions of years, the sea, the air, and the sun are still singing the song we must begin to appreciate once more.

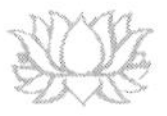

In Practice

The Timeless Way

As long as creation dominates your existence, you will keep growing and evolving. Evolution thwarts entropy, decay, and aging. The most creative people in any field intuitively draw on this understanding. They grow with full consciousness that they are the source of their own power, and whatever their field, certain traits are generally shared by them:

1. They are able to contact and enjoy silence.
2. They connect with and enjoy Nature.
3. They trust their feelings.
4. They can remain centered and function amid confusion and chaos.
5. They are childlike—they enjoy fantasy and play.

6. They self-refer: They place the highest trust in their own consciousness.
7. They are not rigidly attached to any point of view: Although passionately committed to their creativity, they remain open to new possibilities.

These seven points give us a practical standard to measure how creatively our lives are proceeding. The following exercise demonstrates how to develop and strengthen these areas.

Exercise 1: Creative Action Plan

Write out an action plan for the next six months based on the seven qualities of very creative people that we have just discussed. You don't have to squeeze every point into each day—just make a commitment to allow these aspects of your life to emerge more fully.

1. EXPERIENCING SILENCE

First, block out some time to experience silence. Ideally this would mean a short period of meditation (fifteen to thirty minutes) in the morning before you go to work, then a second period just after you get home in the evening. This is a time simply to be, and yet its very simplicity can make it the most important time of your life. Silence is a precious commodity, particularly in the hustle-and-bustle of modern society.

Silence is the great teacher, and to learn its lessons you must pay attention to it.

2. Spending time in Nature

Plan to spend a period of time contacting Nature. There is no healthier way to discharge pent-up energies. The mind-body system throws off its excess energies spontaneously when you remove yourself from the artificial confines of the material world and return to Nature. If you can find a patch of ground to lie down on, shoes off and arms outstretched to the sun, take advantage of it. Short of that, seek out experiences of Nature where you live, stopping for a few moments in the evening to watch the sunset and gaze at the moon and stars.

Even in the heart of congested urban areas, you can tend a windowsill garden so that you can watch a seed grow; walking out onto the roof of your building to absorb the sun also affords some contact with Nature. However you can manage it, capture at least a few moments of freshness and feel the nourishing touch of earth, sun, and sky.

3. Experiencing and trusting emotions

Begin a journal of your feelings. Simply make a list of some key emotions and note *one example* of each as it arises in your day. Start with key words for the basic positive emotions, such as:

love	joy
sympathy	acceptance
happiness	friendliness
trust	compassion

Next, make a column for more abstract feelings associated with creativity and personal growth, such as:

insight	intuition
discovery	transcendence
faith	merging
forgiveness	peace
revelation	

Last, note the primary negative emotions, such as:

anger	envy
anxiety	sorrow
guilt	greediness
distrust	selfishness

Look at this sheet of paper in the morning and take it with you to work as a reminder. Although you will get the most benefit by actually writing down your feelings in some detail, making them explicit and reliving how strong each feeling was, what kind of circumstances triggered it, and how much a particular emotion meant to you, you can do very well with a silent journal. That is, glance down the list and simply remember each emotion briefly. Your goals with this journal are as follows:

1. To discover how often you feel things that get overlooked.
2. To permit the spontaneous release of emotions that you would normally repress or try to forget.
3. To truly know your emotions. This is the first stage of mastering your emotions.
4. To make your emotions enjoyable. The life of feelings is meant to be rich and satisfying, but if your emotions are strangers to you, you cannot enjoy them.

It's important not to focus too much on negative emotions, which are the easiest for everyone to experience and usually are the most self-serving. I ask you to bring up negative emotions so that you may gain insight into their origin.

Being genuinely in touch with emotions tends to be tremendously difficult amid work and other activities. Yet nothing is more important than experiencing your feelings. You are the totality of all the relationships you have, and the most accurate mirror of them is your emotions.

4. Remaining centered amid chaos

In order to remain centered and calm when everything around you is in confusion, you need to develop skills for finding your center. To do that, isolate two times in your workday when things are most hectic and stressful for you. Now plan to take five minutes to center yourself just before these two periods, using the following technique:

Find a place where you can be alone, one that is as quiet as possible. Sit comfortably and close your eyes. Pay attention to your breathing. See the air as faint swirls coming into your nostrils and gently flowing out again. After two minutes, begin to feel your body (i.e., note the sensations inside your body, on your skin, the weight of your limbs, etc.). After a minute, gently bring your attention to the center of your chest and lightly rest it there. Within a few seconds your attention will probably be distracted. Don't resist this, but when you notice what is happening, gently return your focus to your chest. End the exercise by sitting quietly, doing nothing.

Although this is a very simple technique, the discharge of negative energies it produces is often quite dramatic—you can feel a heavy burden lifting off your shoulders and sense a lightness and calm infusing your whole being. Most important, you will begin to experience that being centered is actually the most natural and comfortable way to be in any situation, no matter how hectic.

5. Being childlike

Write down two or three things you can do tomorrow that are totally childlike. Think of something that evokes childhood for you—eating an ice cream cone, being on the playground, playing games with the shapes of clouds. Begin to incorporate these activities more and more into your present life. Your goal is to find that place inside you where you are still a carefree child. Your childhood is still there with you, ready to be evoked and integrated into your being.

What usually happens over time is that we lose track of the joy inside us.

Ultimately, the desire to be young again is a

symbol of the deeper desire to remain new. Babies and young children have no problem with this. By putting yourself back into the most childlike mindset you can imagine, you open the way for learning, as Almaas puts it, that "we are the pleasure, we are the joy, we are the most profound significance and the highest value."

6. BEING SELF-REFERRAL

The highest state of consciousness available to us is unity, which erases the distinction between observer and observed. In unity, everything you once thought was "out there" is seen to be part of yourself. What prevents this experience is a false sense of self built from images of past experience. To get rid of this baggage and reexperience yourself as a free, uncluttered person, you have to work at stripping away the crusted varnish of self-image.

Your action plan can take many different directions in accomplishing this goal.

- You can take up a new activity that is totally incongruous with your self-image. Take up aerobic dancing if you are a gray-flanneled business executive, or weight lifting if you're a housewife. Expose yourself to people and situations that challenge you to grow beyond old habits.

- Write your autobiography. Putting down every detail of your life as candidly and honestly as possible will help you detach from ingrained attitudes by showing you where they came from.
- Resolve to take one step every day to correct some behavior that you know isn't an expression of the real you. For example, you may be an habitual people-pleaser. The next time you find yourself falling into that trap, say what you really feel. On the other hand, if you are always outspoken and tend to feel that others should listen to you, stop yourself and listen to them for a change. These simple exercises can actually be quite challenging; you need to learn to lower your social facade, and the more you practice, the less critical you will find it is to wear the mask.

7. Practicing Nonattachment

To be unattached means that you are free from outside influences that overshadow your real self. This lesson isn't one our culture teaches us. Modern people place a high value on being committed, excited, passionate, deeply involved, and so forth, and they fail to realize that these qualities are not the opposite of nonattachment. To be committed to a relationship, for example, ultimately means to have enough love and understanding to let the other person be who he or she wants to be.

The paradox is that to get the most passion from life, you must be able to stand back and be yourself.

Speaking for myself, I've found that moments of nonattachment are characterized by the following:

- I am present with my body.
- My breathing becomes very refined, approaching stillness.
- Mental activity has calmed down.
- I feel no threat; there is a certainty of belonging.
- I perceive my inner world as an open space with no boundaries; awareness extends in all directions rather than being focused on specific thoughts.
- Self-acceptance flows out into the environment. Things "out there" seem intimate to me, an extension of myself.

This experience of unity is also my working definition of love.

For your action plan to succeed, you need to find an outlet for your love, a place where you can give it freely. Love wants to find itself, and when the circuit is complete, bliss flows. Ask yourself, "Where do I find bliss?" then write down the steps you can take to increase this experience in your life.

Do not confuse pleasure with love. There are many things that give pleasure, such as watching television, with very little love in them. Love certainly brings pleasure but in a more profound way. Carrying a meal to a shut-in is an act of love that is far more pleasurable than watching television, for example, and there is much more to learn from such an action in terms of sharing, compassion, and understanding.

When you make your list, you'll find that many of your most cherished moments of bliss have gone forever. For example, you cannot duplicate the first new feeling of falling in love with the person to whom you are now married. But love has depth after depth. As you make your list, you will remember how you felt the day your children were born, and in that reminder is a clue: Your children can still be a source of bliss, if you resolve to reach deeper into your relationship with them. Nothing is more important than reconnecting with your bliss. Nothing is as rich. Nothing is more real.

Exercise 2: Being Love versus Being in Love

I'd like to explore the state of love further, because it is the surest road back to Being. The ancient sages declared that ultimately everything is made of consciousness, and when we experience consciousness purely, with no extraneous images or assumptions, that is love. The merging of love, truth, and reality is the great revelation of unity consciousness, the moment when a person can truthfully say, "I am the All," and, "I am love," in the same breath.

Being *in* love is not the same state as this. When you fall in love, an opening is created for repressed feelings to rush forth and attach themselves to another person. If the love is deep enough, the other person seems ideal and perfect (this has nothing to do with his or her actual state, which could be quite imperfect and even destructive). But the force of love changes reality by changing the perceiver.

In a series of revealing experiments, Harvard psychologist David C. McClelland probed the physiology of love. He had a group of subjects view a short film of Mother Teresa in her daily work of caring for sick and abandoned children in Calcutta. The film displayed a profound outpouring of love. As the audience watched the film, McClelland discovered that a marker in their immune systems increased—this was SIgA, or salivary immunoglobulin antigen. High levels of SIgA, as measured in people's saliva, indicates a high immune response; as it happens, an elevated immune response is also characteristic of people who have recently fallen in love.

McClelland also found that the positive effect on the viewers' immune response declined and disappeared an hour or two after they had viewed the film. It remained highest among those subjects who reported a strong sense of being loved in their own lives and having strong ties to family and friends. This implied that some people are already in a state conducive to love. Instead of experiencing it as a passing state, they had incorporated it as a trait. In other words, the statement of the enlightened sage, "I am love," was present in these people, if to a smaller degree.

What all this implied to McClelland was that love is a state that transcends reason and whose purpose is simply to allow the experience of a larger shared reality.

This describes a step into the realm of timeless love. When two people use their love for each other as a doorway into this realm, the death of the loved one does not close the door or deprive the other of the flow of love. Ultimately, all love comes from within. We are deluding ourselves when we believe that another person is who we love; the other person is a pretext by which we give ourselves permission to feel love. Only you can open and close your heart. The power of love to nurture and sustain us depends on our commitment to it "in here."

It is important to talk about love, to think about it, to seek it out, and to encourage it. To put this in the form of an exercise, make a commitment to yourself to do the following:

1. Think about love. Take time to recall the love you shared with your parents. Dwell upon what is most lovable about the person who is most loving in your life today. Read deeply the poetry of love, such as is found in Shakespeare's sonnets.

2. Talk about love. Express your feelings directly to someone you love. If you cannot do it verbally, write a letter or a poem. You don't have to send it; the exercise is for you, to stimulate the state of love in every cell. But sending it is preferable, for you want to hear expressions of love in return. Don't let your love be something taken for granted.

3. Seek out love. This is possible in many ways. Intimacy in our society is closely identified with sexual encounters, but it is an act of love to give help to the homeless and the sick, to deliver a

sincere compliment, or to write a note of thanks and praise. People like to hear that they are loved and appreciated, and if you seek out opportunities to fulfill their needs in this area, their gratitude will be mirrored in your physiology as the bliss of being loved in return.

4. Encourage love. As parents we often teach our children that being openly affectionate and loving is appropriate for babies and toddlers but not for anyone older than that. In teaching manners and respect, we often create a gap that love is too sensitive and shy to cross. We inflict this sense of separation on our children because it was inflicted on us. The story of almost everyone is a story of love waiting to be coaxed out, of affection that has to wait in silence because it is afraid to emerge.

So take it as your duty to give those around you permission to love. Encourage their affection by showing it yourself, without regard for what you may get in return. Real love gains complete satisfaction simply by flowing out to what is loved; if love comes back, that is an added joy, but it isn't required or demanded.

The education of love begins in a moment and ends in eternity. It is sparked by feelings of delight and resolves into the peace that belongs to Being itself.

Use love as your mirror of the timeless; let it nurture your certainty that you are beyond change, beyond the memory of yesterday and the dream of tomorrow. There are infinite ways to discover your true Being, but love holds the brightest torch. If you follow it, you will be guided beyond the limits of age and death. Come out of the circle of time and find yourself in the circle of love.

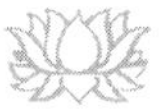

EPILOGUE

TODAY, THE FASTEST GROWING SEGMENT OF THE American population is over the age of 90, and soon it will be over the age of 100. We do not need to be convinced that something dramatic is happening in the biology of aging. Moreover, research continues to show that the biomarkers of aging, such as blood pressure, bone density, body temperature regulation, muscle mass, strength of muscles, the ability to utilize sugar, sex hormone levels, hearing, immune function and near-point vision, can all be improved, even late in life. In other words, the major biomarkers of aging are all reversible. This means aging is *reversible.*

I'm convinced that if you do the exercises in this book, you will dramatically slow down and even reverse the aging process. Remember the basic principles contained in these pages.

1. Aging is reversible. Biological age does not correspond to chronological age. You can be chronologically twenty years old, but if you're emotionally and physically burnt out, your biology will be that of an old person. Or, you can be 70 years old and be physically, emotionally, and spiritually fit and your biology reflects the stamina, the vitality, the creativity, the alertness, and the dynamism of youth.
2. Aging, or entropy, is accelerated by the accumulation of toxins in the body. These toxins occur as a result of a toxic environment, toxicity or contamination in food or drink, toxic relationships, and toxic emotions. Eliminating these toxins will influence your biological clock in the direction of youth.
3. Physical exercise, including weight training, has a direct effect on the biomarkers of aging and will reverse the aging process.
4. Proper nutrition and nutritional supplements, including antioxidants, are a very useful adjunct in slowing down the aging process.

5. Meditation lowers biological age.
6. Love is the most powerful and potent medicine. It heals but it also renews.

Finally what is a timeless mind, and how does it influence the biological clock? More and more, I've become convinced that our experience of time directly influences the activity of such a clock. If you're "running out of time," your biological clock will speed up. If you "have all the time in the world," your biological clock will slow down. In moments of transcendence, when time stands still, your biological clock will stop. The spirit is that domain of our awareness where there's no time. Time is the continuity of memory, which uses the ego as an internal reference point. When we go beyond our ego and enter the realm of our spirit, we break the barrier of time. Ultimately, both the quality and quantity of life depend on our sense of identity. If we have meaning and purpose in our lives and our identity is not tied to "a skin-encapsulated ego," then both the quality and quantity of life will be dramatically enhanced. More than any nutritional supplement or exercise, the most important thing that you can do to change your life is to practice the following principles:

- Have your attention on the timeless, the eternal, the infinite.

- Get your ego out of the way.
- Be natural; relinquish the need to hide constantly behind a social mask.
- Surrender to the mystery of the universe.
- Have a sense of communion with Spirit or Divinity.
- Be defenseless, relinquishing the need to defend your point of view.

I wish you good luck with your journey of life.

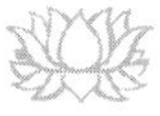

About the Author

DEEPAK CHOPRA is the author of more than fifty books translated in over thirty-five languages, including numerous *New York Times* bestsellers in both the fiction and nonfiction categories. Chopra's Wellness Radio airs weekly on Sirius Stars, Channel 102, which focuses on the areas of success, love, sexuality and relationships, well being, and spirituality. He is founder and president of the Alliance for a New Humanity and can be contacted at www.deepakchopra.com. *Time* magazine heralds Deepak Chopra as one of the top 100 heroes and icons of the century, and credits him as "the poet-prophet of alternative medicine." (June 1999).

Enjoy these new bestsellers by Deepak Chopra

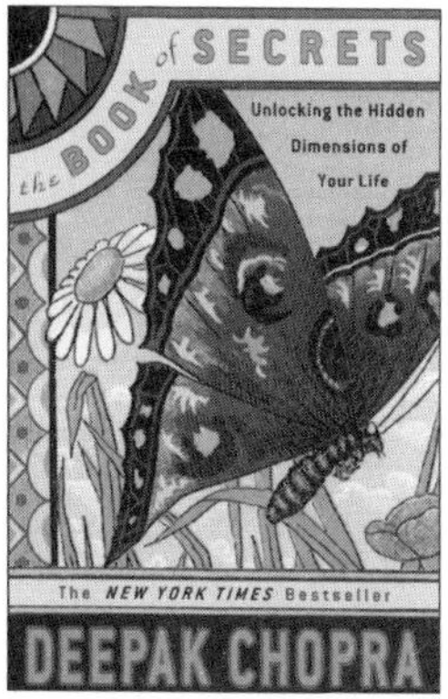

The Book of Secrets
Unlocking the Hidden Dimensions of Your Life
978-1-4000-9834-7
$14.95 paper (Canada: $19.95)

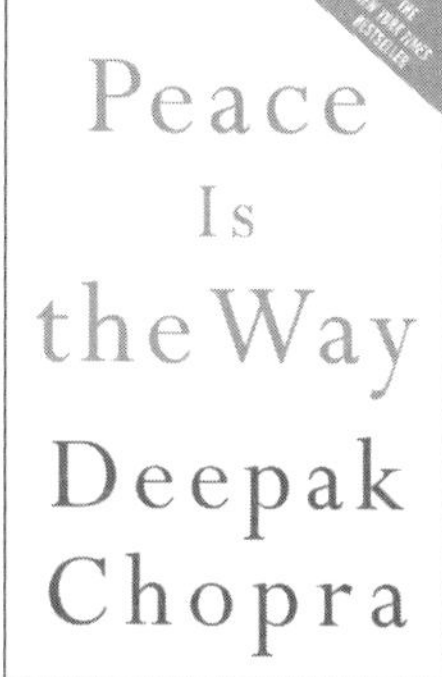

Peace Is the Way
Bringing War and Violence to an End
978-0-307-33981-2
$13.00 paper (Canada: $18.00)

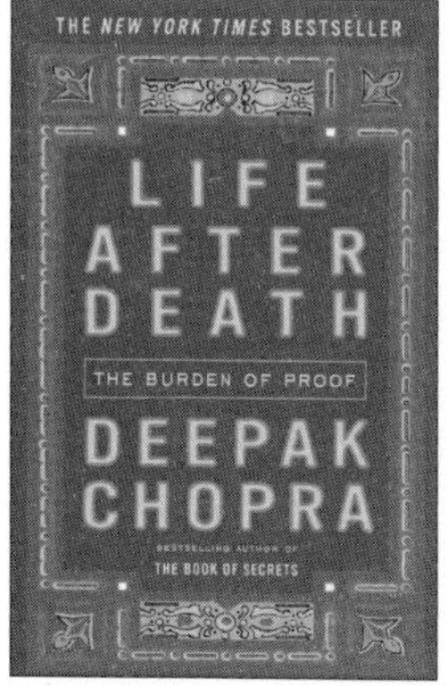

Life After Death
The Burden of Proof
978-0-307-34578-3
$24.00 hardcover (Canada: $32.00)

Available wherever books are sold.

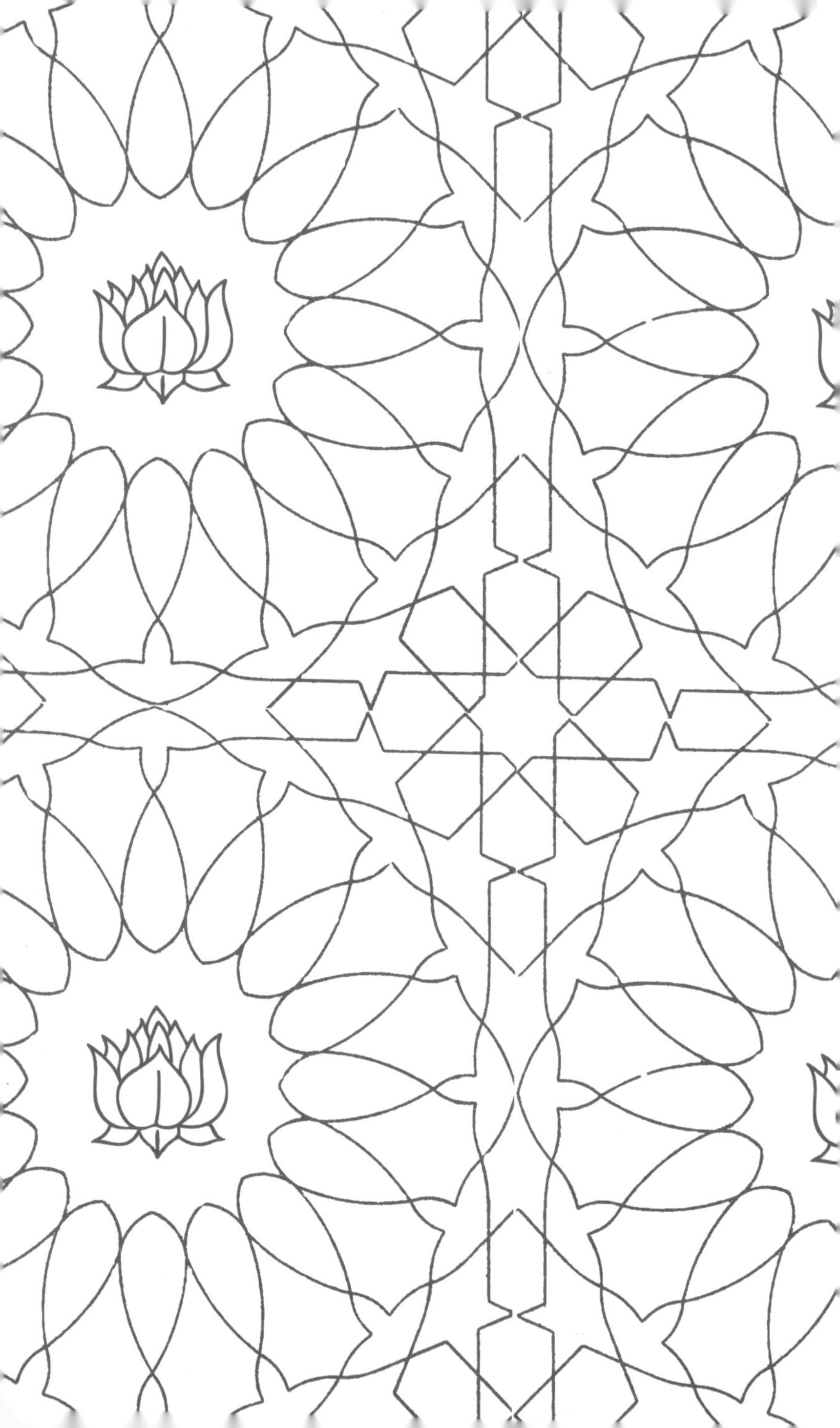